Lifeline to Care with Dignity

Caring for the Memory Impaired

Kathie T. Erwin, Ph.D., Ed.D.

)7

'3 blications

'g, Florida

A Note to the Reader

All case examples used for illustrative purposes in this text are based on fictionalized characters, and imply no reference to actual persons. While every effort has been made to provide up-to-date information regarding Alzheimer's disease and other memory impairment difficulties, neither Caremor Publications nor the author can guarantee the accuracy of the information with reference to ongoing research and new insights into these complex issues. Also, this publication has been designed to provide accurate and authoritative information in regard its subject matter. It is sold with the understanding that the publisher is not engaged in rendering legal or other professional services. If legal advice or other expert assistance is required, the reader should seek the services of a competent professional person.

Wellness Facilitator^{SM} *is a service mark of Caremor Corporation*

Publisher's Cataloging-in-Publication
(Provided by Quality Books, Inc.)

Erwin, Kathie T., 1950-
    Lifeline to care with dignity : caring for the memory impaired /
Kathie T. Erwin ; [edited by Annette Martino]. -- 1st ed.
    p. cm.
    Includes bibliographical references and index.
    ISBN: 1-887454-01-2

    1. Memory disorders--Patients--Nursing home care.   2. Memory
disorders--Patients--Home care. 3. Nursing assessment. 4. Nursing
care plans. 5. Home nursing. I. Title.

RC350.5.E79 1997   610.73'68
                           QBI97-40755

Printed in the United States of America
Caremor Publications
25 Second Street North
St. Petersburg, FL 33701
(813) 894-5333

"Dr. Erwin has written a much needed guide for both professional and family caregivers of the memory impaired. Professionals will profit from her system for assessing memory loss and her excellent guidance on communication with the memory impaired, modifying the residential environment, behavior management, and enabling staff to become 'wellness' facilitators. Family caregivers will find that she has translated her professional insights into language that can be easily understood. For the families who provide the vast majority of elder care in America, this outstanding work is truly a 'lifeline.'"

Thelma E. Bland
Commissioner
Department for the Aging
Commonwealth of Virginia

"The down-to-earth approach to sophisticated ideas and concepts makes this book readable ... a text which offers excellent humanistic skills necessary to promote the welfare of Alzheimer's and other memory impaired patients ... for both professional caregivers and family members."

Shanta Sharma, Ph.D.
Professor
Henderson State University, Arkadelphia, AR

"As both a professional caregiver for the past 25 years and a family caregiver, I believe one's perception of the memory impaired as well as one's view of caregiving are basic to success as a caregiver ... (this book) provides caregivers with the understanding, techniques, and strategies needed to provide love, dignity, and feelings of satisfaction to memory impaired older adults."

R. Nacken Gugel, Ph.D.
Clinical Psychologist
Lynn University, Miami, FL

Dedication

To my mother in law, Edythe Parker Barnett,
who at her 90th birthday, is aging with style.

Contents

Acknowledgements   *vi*

Foreward   *vii*

Preface   *ix*

1   What is Memory Impairment?   1

2   Stages of Memory Impairment   15

3   Assessment of the Memory Impaired Adult   29

4   A Basic Assessment System   43

5   Communication   63

6   Modifying the Environment for the Memory Impaired   75

7   Managing Difficult Behaviors   93

8   Memory Impairment is a Family Issue   113

9   Stress: the Caregiver's Constant Companion   135

10   When Caregiving Staff Become Wellness Facilitators   151

Glossary   *171*

References   *175*

Index   *181*

Acknowledgments

The author extends grateful appreciation to:

Annette Martino, Executive Editor, whose vision for "Facilitating Wellness" is the cornerstone of this book. With the expertise of 25 years in elder care and her passion to raise the consciousness of caregivers who provide direct services to memory impaired persons, Ms. Martino's work is influential in today's health care delivery systems. As founder and president of Caremor Corporation, she has made the commitment to share the Caremor philosophy of "Facilitating Wellness" with family and facility caregivers through this book and with an additional series of related publications for future release.

Dr. Bert Erwin, my husband, and our twin daughters, **Robin** and **Kelly,** who take on extra responsibilities and offer encouragement each time Mom writes a book.

Senior Meadows of St. Petersburg, Florida for welcoming the photo team to their attractive facility near the downtown waterfront.

Cover models, **Thelma Simpson** and **Aleyda Peters,** who genuinely represent the positive caregiving relationship.

Ken Kinzel, whose creative touch is evident in the cover photo and format for the text.

Jan Ladd, RN, MA and **Marty Johnson** for their efforts in arranging the cover photography and coordinating with the Caremor program at Senior Meadows.

Foreword

As our society continues to age, one of the most pressing problems we face is the care of our impaired persons. Among the most vexing of these impairments are those of memory and memory-related behaviors. The care of memory impaired persons represents a great social challenge, as it touches on yet uncharted territory, where the tools and techniques for dignified care are only now in development and their validation and broad application are not yet complete. It is with this in mind that Dr. Kathie T. Erwin has written a comprehensive guide for the care of the memory impaired person.

Herein Dr. Erwin describes in a concise and user-friendly manner, her thoughts on the tools and techniques for memory-related behavioral assessment and the dignified management of the impaired person. Dr. Erwin uses real-life examples to document the problems faced in recognizing memory impairments and their related behavioral problems, then takes the reader through a series of steps to deal with these problems. The novel process used in this guide keeps the individual's dignity as the top priority at each stage of the diagnosis and compassionate care. This is important, as impaired individuals are too often treated as subjects of our efforts to provide care, rather than as persons whose quality of life is improved by their participation in the process of the provision of care.

Sometime during our lives, most of us will be faced with the care of an impaired person, whether that person be us or a loved one. I hope the guide provided in this text will be used broadly, and the techniques proposed herein will be tested, validated, improved upon and applied to the compassionate care of our memory impaired loved ones. They deserve the best care we can provide.

James W. Simpkins, Ph.D.
The Frank A. Duckworth Professor of
Drug Discovery and Director,
Center for the Neurobiology of Aging
University of Florida, Gainesville, Florida

Preface

Ask a group of older adults to name their greatest fears about aging and the most common responses are "going to live in a nursing home" and "losing memory due to Alzheimer's disease." Those are critical life change issues that begin casually with forgetfulness and become severe enough to steal away independence. For many individuals and their families, memory impairment moves from being an inconvenience or embarrassment to a cause of significant changes for the family in relationships, finances and emotional stress. Reaching families and caregivers who deal with the impact of memory impairment is the heart of this text.

As memory loss progresses, the confused and memory impaired person deals with the double trauma of losing a connection with the past through memories and leaving a familiar home environment. No matter how loving or respectful the care is in a nursing home or assisted living facility, it is still being provided in a strange environment.

To gain an appreciation of how strange are the changes that memory impairment imposes, imagine driving home one evening and being kidnapped by Martians. The Martians speak to you, but you can't understand their language and they can't understand your words. Suddenly you arrive at a nice looking home with several other earth people. It seems pleasant, no one is unkind, but it's not home. The Martians try to get you to sing songs and play games. You just want to go home. They ask you to swallow odd looking liquids and take showers that are too hot or too cold. Some of the Martians seem to care about you while others barely pay any attention as they go about their tasks. Just when you begin to recognize some words you overhear two Martians speaking as if you are not there and announcing that you will never go back to your earth home again. They tell you that this is home. You may not know how to unlock the door or find your clothes, but you know for certain that this is absolutely not home! What feelings might surface at such an experience?

Confusion? Disorientation? Anger? Fear? Loneliness? Despair? Perhaps all these feelings surface with overwhelming force creating a disastrous result.

Family and staff caregivers may not be able to literally "walk a mile in the shoes" of a memory impaired person. However, caregivers can be respectful of the feelings that are a very real part of the day-to-day life of the memory impaired person. Being forgetful does not imply that a person is without feelings. Neither are caregivers without feelings when dealing with the often difficult behaviors and profound needs of caring for memory impaired persons.

Lifeline to Care with Dignity serves as an advocate for facilitating wellness in the care of memory impaired adults by teaching this concept to family and staff caregivers.

1

What is Memory Impairment?

Basic definition of memory

Abnormal memory functioning

What causes confusion and memory impairment?

When forgetfulness leads to confusion

Forgetting a phone number, misplacing the car keys, or mixing up the numbers in a mailing address are odd things that happen to people of all ages. Young and middle age adults tend to laugh at and easily dismiss these "OOPS" experiences. Life in a computerized world exposes people to a flood of information from the Internet, e-mail, television, radio, newspapers, and magazines. No wonder that "information overload" causes stress and memory recall problems even among college students.

Older adults nearing traditional retirement age (62 to 65) take a far more serious view of memory problems. The early phase of memory impairment is difficult to distinguish from age-related memory decline. Thus the fear of becoming memory impaired is very real among older adults. Many seniors are reluctant to accept the typical age-related changes in memory as a normal part of aging.

An example of this reluctance is Edna, who didn't want to get professional advice and risk hearing bad news about her husband, George. Even after retirement as an engineering designer, George spent hours constructing elaborate model airplanes. Gradually he lost interest, broke parts and became angry trying to read the directions. Edna's way of helping George stay mentally sharp was to demand that he complete the daily newspaper word search and crossword puzzle. If he failed to meet her demand, she resorted to holding his lunch as hostage until he completed his task. No puzzles, no lunch. What happened more often than not was that he wandered around mumbling angry words and ignoring the puzzle.

Edna's well meaning efforts did nothing to delay the progression of George's memory impairment. Her approach to helping his memory was to demand performance rather than challenge George's skills. She also failed to consider the negative effects of hunger, frustration and fatigue that compromise mental performance for persons of any age.

The burden of frequent forgetfulness weighs heavily on the older person as safety and health are compromised. The most common motions of living become difficult to complete . Even chores that have been repeated thousands of times over the past forty or fifty years seem strange.

Seventy year old Gwen has lived alone for twenty years since her husband died. Always a wonderful housekeeper, she is upset about "never getting my house in order." Every morning she begins to make the bed, becomes bewildered halfway through the process, then wanders away in distress. Later while cooking dinner, Gwen forgets that the eggs just finished boiling and reaches into the still hot water to get an egg. The next day when a neighbor asks how such a terrible burn occurred on the hand, Gwen looks at the scar as if she never saw it before and does not remember what happened.

As forgetfulness and confusion result in a danger to an older person's safety or health, the likely culprits are memory impairment or other physical and psychological conditions.

What is Memory?

Memories are the subject of songs, poems and books. Memories of home, family, children, friends, lovers, and travel are like favorite movies played in the mind for personal pleasure. Human beings value memories as part of their life stories and a reminder of their heritage from past generations. Being able to recall information learned years or months ago can be applied to present tasks. Or, as with George, the inability to recall spelling and vocabulary made crossword puzzles impossible to complete. Memories are also reminders of how to handle practical, everyday tasks such as taking a bath, getting dressed, folding the clothes, and dialing the telephone. Edna did not remember that the water on the stove had just completed boiling. The day after she burned herself by reaching in the water, she did not recall how the injury happened. Her ability to manage this basic cooking technique, which she has done hundreds of times in her life, suggests a memory problem that goes beyond simple forgetfulness.

The technical and medical explanations of how all the pathways and connections in the brain function are very complex. This text is more interested in supporting a working understanding of the memory processes of the human brain so that persons with various levels of training will find this information useful and practical. By choice, the longer, more precise medical terminology is translated into concepts that focus our attention on the person with memory impairment rather than the disease (or medical model) orientation that focuses on the impairment.

Basic definition of memory: a process of receiving information, storing information, and retrieving information. The two types of memory are short-term memory and long-term memory.

Short-term memory is the active process that operates in the here and now. As information is received, it goes first to the short-term memory. With so many distractions in daily living (i.e., radio, television, billboards, nearby conversations), a lot of information passes through the short-term memory without being stored. Think about looking up a telephone number in the yellow pages. Most people repeat the number over and over before dialing. Perhaps you have stood at a telephone booth fumbling to find a quarter while whispering the number "123-4567, 123-4567." Keeping that number active in your mind was smart because short-term memory is very short. Information received into the short term memory and not acted upon is lost in thirty seconds or less. Now you know why it's so easy to forget the name of a new person after being introduced. Short-term memory is a "use-it-or-lose-it" process.

The capacity for short-term memory is not as great as that for long-term memory. Think of short-term memory as one or two sentence notes written on a 3 x 5 index card. When the card is filled, no more information can be added. Some sentences can be erased to make room to write new information. Since a file card can be easily lost or misplaced, the information needs to be recorded in a more appropriate place. All or part of the information on that card can be re-written on a calendar, grocery list, or diary for future reference. Information stored for future retrieval becomes part of the long-term memory. Once the information is stored or eliminated as not necessary, the short-term memory is open to new input.

Available space in the short-term memory is limited and relatively small as illustrated by the space on a blank 3x5 index card. The limitations of short-term memory exist for everyone, regardless of age, intelligence, or education. If the information received into the short-term memory is important, it must pass to the next stage for storage.

Long-term memory is the permanent storage center with unlimited capacity. Storing information and retrieving information occurs in the long-term memory. How effectively information can be located within the long-term memory depends on how well it was coded and stored. Think of looking up information about travel in an encyclopedia. Like long-term memory, an encyclopedia holds a vast amount of information that is carefully coded (labeled) by alphabetical order, topic, and related topics. A poorly coded encyclopedia or other reference book would still contain necessary information but make it too difficult and frustrating to be useful.

Safely storing information in the long-term memory begins in the short-term memory. During those seconds after information is received into the short-term memory, an effort must be made to repeat and code the information for storage in the long-term memory. The better the coding system, the better the chances of easy retrieval. Much like the average home storage closet; keeping linens, luggage, holiday decorations, etc. in labeled boxes or on shelves with similar items is the easiest way to organize and locate items. Overstuff that closet with no organization and items are quickly hidden and lost.

Try to overstuff the short-term memory and information gets lost, pushed out to make room for more.

Although sweeping the floor and fixing cereal for breakfast are done in the "here and now," the information is merely passing through short-term memory. The information for those ordinary, repeated actions was recalled from the long-term memory as needed. The long-term memory is a "how to" manual for activities of daily living. Calling up information from the long-term memory is how we know the way to fold the laundry, go to the bathroom, get dressed, and dial the telephone.

The Information Processing Network

Incoming information is first "caught" by the short-term or working memory. If it is important or interesting to an individual, information can be "taught" to the long-term or remote memory through a personal system of coding for storage. Retrieving the information from long-term memory into a completed "thought" happens faster with a good coding system. Within the normal aging process, a decline occurs in the capacity of the short-term memory as well as the speed or amount of information recalled from the long-term memory (Lovelace, 1990). Taken alone, that statement may lead to an ageist conclusion. Remember: All older people are not forgetful. However, due to physical aging, the potential for forgetfulness increases.

Abnormal Memory Functioning

At any point in the memory process that a breakdown occurs, the result is abnormal (or less than normal) memory functioning. This condition may be temporary or permanent. Temporary memory problems can be the result of medication, anesthesia, depression, extreme fatigue, nutritional deficiencies, sensory deficits, medical conditions, or grief (loss of relationship or death of a loved one). Change these causal factors and the memory problems disappear or diminish significantly. Permanent memory problems are chronic with potentially increasing loss of memory due to circumstances such as head injury, chemical poisoning, or a type of dementia. The causal factors of permanent conditions cannot be reversed, so the conditions tend to worsen over time.

Stated in simple terms, breakdown in the memory process is evident in three types of abnormal memory functioning.

1. Persistent problems with short-term memory.
An older adult may easily recall her social security number and birthdates of a dozen grandchildren yet forget what she is doing in the middle of preparing dinner. The problem is particularly notable when the short-term memory loss happens regardless of whether the person is tired or rested, hungry or satisfied, sick or well.

2. Difficulty storing into long-term memory.
Another older person struggles with learning to use the remote control for a new television. Even though a neighbor patiently explains and demonstrates which buttons to push to change channels, the confused person can only mimic the actions using short-term memory. Somewhere a breakdown in coding and storage processes prevents the new information from being stored in long-term memory for use at another time.

3. Difficulty retrieving from long-term memory.
An older person may have only limited access to information stored in the long-term memory. For example, the older person recalls vivid details about a lesson learned in elementary school, but cannot remember the steps to complete a craft learned several months ago. Long-term memory retrieval problems are like a stuck file drawer. Access to the information in the stuck drawer is restricted while permitting access to information in the other drawers.

Breakdowns in the memory process are often described as "confusion" or "memory impairment" as if the words are interchangeable. Although both terms refer to problems with memory functioning, the difference is significant.

Confusion is an interruption of the memory process resulting in temporary or episodic disorientation sufficient to cause difficulty functioning within the environment.

The degree and extent of confusion varies among persons. In some cases, a reversal of the causal factors restores functioning. For example, an older person suffering extreme nutritional deficiencies may appear very confused. After that person's nutritional balance improves and physical strength returns to pre-illness status, signs of confusion are gone. This situation is totally different from persons whose confusion is linked to irreversible brain cell damage.

Memory Impairment is a chronic interruption of the memory process resulting in permanent disorientation to person, place and time that is evidenced by a progressive decline in short-term and long-term memory.

At this point in medical research, memory impairments caused by disease or other damage to brain cells is irreversible. What makes these conditions even more troublesome is that the memory loss does not happen and then freeze at that point of loss. The memory functioning continues to decline in either a steady or intermittent manner until death.

What Causes Confusion and Memory Impairment?

Determining the exact causes of confusion and memory impairment is not clear in all situations. Certain factors have known relationships to some types of memory impairment. Other factors still unknown by medical research are like a mystery waiting to be solved.

The following chart contains a summary of the commonly encountered conditions that can lead to memory impairment.

Reversible Conditions	Irreversible Conditions
Depression	Alzheimer's Disease
Anesthesia	Vascular Dementia
Medication	HIV related Dementia
Extreme Fatigue	Other Dementias
Nutritional Deficiencies	Head Injury
Sensory Deficits	Chemical Poisoning
Medical Conditions	
Grief	

Reversible Conditions

Depression as a single episode or a recurrent problem is a pervasive disturbance of mood with feelings of helplessness and hopelessness. Under the cloud of depression, a formerly cheerful, positive person can become anxious, withdraw from social activities, and develop irrational fears about safety, illness or death. A severely depressed person may claim to see things not present (delusions) or have physical pain that cannot be diagnosed. Depression is one of the most common emotional problems of older adults (Butler, Lewis and Sunderland, 1991).

Recognizing depression as a serious problem among nursing home residents is important for caregivers. According to the National Institutes of Health (1991) nearly one out óf every four nursing home residents (15 - 25 percent) experiences depression. That is greater than the 15 percent of older persons living within the community who are depressed. Even after treatment, "13 percent of nursing home residents develop a new episode of major depression over a one year period, and another 18 percent develop new depressive symptoms" (NIH, 1991, p. 8).

This author recalls a disturbing experience in asking a physician to consider treating depressive symptoms in an older adult nursing home resident. The symptoms were dismissed by the physician in a chart note: "of course she's depressed, she's old and lives in a nursing home, what do you expect?" Such an ageist attitude was certainly not expected from a physician who regularly treats nursing home residents. Approximately 70 percent of depressed older adults improve with treatment (Hinrichsen, 1992).

Anesthesia for minor or major surgery frequently requires a longer period of complete recuperation for older adults than for younger adults. Stories abound of the spouse who "doesn't act like" himself or herself after elective surgery or anesthesia to set broken bones due to an accidental fall. During the immediate recovery period, the older adult may be very disoriented and unable to remember even basic personal information (i.e., date of birth, home address or adult children's married names). As the drug wears off and the healing processes of the body begin to restore physical health, the emotional confusion gives way to pre-anesthesia levels of functioning.

Medication that heals can also harm if taken incorrectly. Many older persons take a variety of prescription and over-the-counter drugs for both ongoing (i.e., high blood pressure, thyroidism) and temporary problems (i.e., upset stomach, cough). Far too many people of all ages fail to recognize that even cold capsules, diuretics, sleep aids and other over-the-counter medications are "drugs." As a result, physicians are at a real disadvantage making prescription decisions without being fully informed of other "drugs" used by their patients.

The risk increases as prescription drugs and the over-the-counter drugs mix in serious and potentially deadly chemical reactions. Harmful side effects include confusion, memory loss, hallucinations, disorientation, paranoia, and anxiety. An older person experiencing a drug reaction is easily mistaken as being memory impaired or psychotic. The medication mixing problem takes longer to discover when that person lives alone or takes drugs not known to the caregiver. As adults age, levels of medication tolerance change, making it difficult to balance a positive effect under ideal conditions. Add even the slightest error or mixing of medications and the danger escalates for older adults.

Extreme fatigue causes persons of any age to be less alert, efficient, or self-aware. Incidents of industrial and traffic accidents increase sharply for persons who are not properly rested. For older adults, extreme fatigue can easily result from caregiving tasks, as well as from various sleep disorders, medication imbalance, television addiction, or emotional distress. Everyone's body needs a certain amount of sleep; not just sleep, but quality sleep in which the body systems are relaxed and refreshed for the next day. Like the old warning about the dangers of "burning the candle at both ends," before long the candle is burned out.

"Burnout" is a popular term for extreme fatigue that affects younger adults who are overworked with jobs and family responsibilities. However, burnout is not a problem reserved for younger adults. Burnout is increasingly found among older adults. With physical exhaustion comes forgetfulness, disorientation, anxiety, confusion, and high risk for accidents. Younger adults with those symptoms are told to "take a cruise" or "move to the country" and "live a less stressful lifestyle." Older adults are more likely to be labeled "confused" and memory impaired" than to be encouraged to take a cruise or get extra help with home or daily care needs.

Nutritional deficiencies are underrated in their potential to cause confusion and memory problems for older adults. Several years ago a local newspaper revealed the tragic story of an older man who was placed under legal guardianship for what the examiners deemed an inability to function due to Alzheimer's disease. His property was sold, including his personal possessions. Within months of receiving a proper diet, socialization and moderate exercise, the older man was fully alert and very angry at how his life had been invaded by strangers. He hired an attorney and fought back. His story is a classic example of how nutritional deficiencies mistakenly appear to be confusion or memory impairment. Older adults whose diet lacks sufficient amounts of B-12, folate, thiamine, and iron are at greater risk for nutritional deficiencies that mimic symptoms of confusion and memory impairment.

Sensory deficits may result from loss or diminished abilities in any of the five senses (touch, taste, smell, hearing, vision). Losing sensory input in later years demands rapid adjustment to new ways of doing familiar tasks. A lack of taste or smell causes a good cook to suddenly seem to lose the ability to prepare food or to complain about foods prepared by other people. Without sensory input from touch, so many ordinary actions become awkward and difficult. Vision and hearing loss create even more problems as older persons lose these familiar means of navigating within the environment.

The disorientation, slowness, anxiety, and fear resulting from sensory losses can mistakenly look like early stages of confusion or memory impairment. Therapeutic options for sensory deficits can be as basic as new eyeglasses, hearing aid, visual or tactical cues in the home, TDD (Telecommunications Device for the Deaf) added to the telephone, closed captioned television, and/or medications. Other options for complex sensory deficits are skill retraining, mobility training, cataract or glaucoma surgery, guide dog, audio books and newspapers, and Braille writing.

Medical conditions are chronic or periodic disorders affecting parts of the body in ways that can alter thought processes and memory.

When the body is out of balance in one area, all systems are compromised. Confusion, memory impairment, and erratic behaviors occur in many persons with metabolic conditions such as thyroidism (i.e., Graves disease), hypoglycemia (low blood sugar), hypoxia (inadequate oxygen to body tissue), hypothermia (abnormally low body temperature), or food allergies.

Grief is a normal response to a deeply felt loss. Mourning the loss of a loved one or friend is a grief response that is generally well understood. Genuine grief is also felt by older persons at the loss of eyesight or hearing, mobility, health, independence, pets, selling the family home, or ceasing a favorite activity (i.e., bridge group, gardening, driving). During the depth of the grieving process, so much emotional energy is centered in the pain that less energy is available for other cognitive requirements. The symptoms of grief and depression are very similar. For example, a grieving person often neglects self-care, fails to eat properly, withdraws from social occasions, speaks about self as being helpless and hopeless, sees everything as negative, and has a short attention span with poor concentration.

Irreversible Conditions

Alzheimer's Disease is the most common form of dementia (loss of mental and cognitive abilities). Approximately fifty diseases are categorized as types of dementia. A person with Alzheimer's disease experiences a steady decline in cognitive processing necessary for abstract and rational thinking, progressive memory loss, difficulty with spoken or written language, decreased impulse control, and loss of social skills. The symptoms are common, yet very unique. Memory loss may be sudden and minimize access to major segments of life memories for one older person while long-term memory loss in another older person is more gradual.

A first time visitor to a nursing home is often surprised at how "healthy and active" residents are when given appropriate activities. Nursing staff know those tense moments when a physically fit Alzheimer's patient makes a dash for an unlocked door. A family caregiver encounters the same concern trying to redirect the Alzheimer's afflicted spouse who is bored and walks briskly out the front door to "go out for a little stroll."

As with other types of dementia, persons with Alzheimer's (particularly in the early stages) do not "look sick." By present medical knowledge, Alzheimer's disease is incurable and progressive over two to twenty years with an average span of ten years prior to death. The care needs of the person with Alzheimer's are also progressively more demanding.

Vascular dementia, formerly known as *multi-infarct dementia*, is actually a series of mini-strokes (or infarcts) that cause damage to areas of the brain. If Alzheimer's disease is like sliding down a slide, then vascular dementia is like falling off a series of cliff ledges. The condition levels out for a period, then falls to another ledge (or level) after a mini-stroke. Changes in functioning are rapid rather than the slow progressive declines of Alzheimer's disease.

Along with the confusion and disorientation, persons with vascular dementia also have loss of useful language, mood swings, trembling and balance problems. The symptoms are variable depending on which area of the brain is affected by each mini-stroke episode.

HIV-related dementia is an outcome of the effects of HIV (human immunodeficiency virus) on the central nervous system. This type of dementia is characterized by forgetfulness, poor concentration, depressed mood, social isolation, and possible delusions or hallucinations.

Other Dementias are outcomes of various diseases which are combined due to the common outcome. Parkinson's disease, Cruetzfeldt-Jakob's disease, Huntington's disease, and Pick's disease are directly linked to the respective diseases with the common characteristics of confusion, memory impairment, and progressive, irreversible decline of cognition.

Head injury or "Dementia Pugilistica" is not often discussed in dealing with dementia since the incidents are vastly fewer than instances of dementia from Alzheimer's or multi-infarct conditions. Similar to multi-infarct dementia, the dementia symptoms from a head injury are related to the areas of the brain that are damaged by impact.

Chemical poisoning is an increasing problem in industrialized countries. As more dangerous chemicals for weapons, construction and energy production are produced and stored, workers and ordinary citizens can unknowingly be in harm's way. An example of chemical poisoning is *Anoxia*, a dementia-like condition that is triggered by carbon-monoxide poisoning.

A Memory Refresher

While reading this chapter, the reader has had to continually code and shift important information from short-term (working) memory to long-term (remote) memory. Gaining any useful information from this chapter is impossible without the ability to receive the information, code information for storage and recall codes to retrieve information when needed. That's the memory process. Get your short-term memory ready to make the shift to long-term as you read this key concept.

Basic definition of memory: a process of receiving information, storing information and retrieving information.

By contrast, memory impairment is abnormal (or less than normal) memory functioning that may be temporary or permanent.

2

Stages of Memory Impairment

Stages of memory impairment

A view of life inside stages 2 - 7

Neurological symptoms of memory impairment

Behavioral and psychological symptoms of memory impairment

Concept of Stages to Define Memory Impairment

Alzheimer's disease, multi-infarct dementia and other types of dementia are irreversible conditions that progressively steal the memory and functioning ability of the victims. Even facing such a formidable obstacle as dementia, the future is not totally bleak. Informed, compassionate caregivers know how to preserve the dignity, abilities, and the simple pleasures of life for the memory impaired.

Exactly what can be done to assist the memory impaired resident with activities of daily living depends on the cognitive abilities that remain. As previously stated, memory impairment is a progressive condition. The only unknown is to what degree and over what period of time an individual with dementia will lose cognitive functioning. In an effort to define the progression of dementia, various theories attempt to track "stages" from confusion to memory impairment. These stages are merely benchmarks to guide the caregiver and family member in understanding how to best work with the remaining skills and growing needs of the memory impaired.

Toward a Balanced View of Stages

The concept of stages is not intended to categorize or typecast in a negative way. One of the important things that is widely accepted about memory impairment is that it is not a "one-size-fits-all" condition. The progression of memory impairment and the skills retained at various points along the decline are unique to each individual. Thus, stages of memory impairment assist health care professionals and caregivers with a frame of reference to use in their evaluation and communication about memory impaired residents.

Applying stages can be even more complex with the rapid changes brought on by the mini-strokes that occur with multi-infarct dementia. With this condition, the cognitive functioning loss can appear to jump around between the stages due to the area of the brain affected by the mini-stroke. Sudden and dramatic cognitive changes (as well as skipping stages) can be found with dementia due to chemical poisoning or head injury. Add in depression, grief, nutritional deficiencies, or any of the reversible conditions to an irreversible dementia and the resident may seem to be in a later stage. Treat the reversible condition and the resident does not "recover" from a later dementia stage, but rather resumes activity closer to the actual stage of the memory impairment.

Regardless of whether you accept the theory of three, four, or seven stages of confusion and memory impairment, all caregivers (family members and health care providers) must understand the limitations of this concept. No matter how well researched, every stage theory needs a warning label:

Stages may become a self-fulfilling prophecy that unintentionally causes caregivers to discourage the remaining abilities of the memory impaired.

When caregivers are rushed or impatient, the temptation is strong to take over and complete those tasks that are performed more slowly by a memory impaired person. For example, a resident may be able to get dressed with calm, step-by-step directions. A family caregiver who is also trying to get the children ready for school or a facility caregiver with six more residents to dress becomes impatient and takes over and completes the job, as if dressing a doll. Every time the caregiver treats the resident as being incapable, the more incapable the resident becomes in all areas. Psychologists call this "learned helplessness;" treating a person as if he or she is helpless discourages independence and results in helpless responses. In a facility, three residents at a certain stage may be unable to dress without significant assistance. But the fourth resident at the same dementia stage takes pleasure in getting dressed with assistance. Individuality prevails even in dementia.

Keeping in mind the cautions of labeling and learned helplessness, let's turn attention back to the positive uses of defining stages. Experienced health care providers apply the concept of stages as background for developing care plans. Although decisions about whether a resident is at "mild" or "moderate" stage of memory impairment is somewhat subjective, it still provides a means of communication necessary among health care providers. These commonly understood definitions are as important in communication among health care providers as standard diagnostic terms are in medicine and psychology. The history of psychology records times before common diagnostic terminology when people were committed to institutions on such practices as one psychiatrist's personal interpretation of ink blots or another psychiatrist's determination of mental illness based on interviews of relatives without ever talking with the patient. To avoid such scary and opinionated diagnostic determinations, sets of symptoms are identified with certain disorders as well as stages of those symptoms which are often identified as "mild, moderate, or severe."

The relevance of stages and other diagnostic definitions seems appropriate for health care providers, but what about family caregivers? For the non-professional or para-professional caregiver, stages are basic road signs to help understand the skills levels in which the memory impaired person functions. Typically, family caregivers have no prior experience with memory impairment. Some idea of progression, even an imperfect one, is better than having no idea of what may happen next. Identifying behaviors and symptoms of progressive stages also relieves family caregivers of guilt or blame being carried for the skill declines seen in the memory impaired person.

Global Deterioration Scale

The Global Deterioration Scale was developed by Reisberg, Ferris, Leon, & Crook, 1982 as a means of defining the stages or levels of disease progression for persons with memory impairment. Professional, para-professional and family caregivers need to be sensitive to the inappropriate use of these stages as "labels." Just as it is dehumanizing to refer to the "Anxiety disorder in Room 123" or the "Kidney dialysis in recovery," it is equally unacceptable to label a person with memory impairment as "acting just like a typical 3rd stager."

Families communicating with other families in support groups also are cautioned to avoid making comparisons between their memory impaired relative and what is heard about the progression or decline of other memory impaired persons. Comparisons often lead to dissatisfaction, guilt and faulty conclusions. Such comparisons can be misused as a basis for generating sympathy; "my relative is sicker than your relative". Stages of dementia progression are most useful in care planning and behavior management where the attention is on quality of life with consideration for limitations. Memory impaired persons are never "stages" or "diagnoses"; they are people who deserve the respect of caregivers and family.

A View of Life Inside Stages 2 - 7

Mary: Stage 2   Very Mild Cognitive Decline

"I'd lose my head if it wasn't attached to my body," Mary explains when she apologizes to the bridge club for being late again. She says she forgot to look at the newsletter with directions to the host home. Later, after leaving the bridge club, Mary picks up her granddaughter at middle school. She talks with a young mother that is familiar, but she can't remember the woman's name. On the way home her granddaughter says, "Gran, you called Mrs. Green, 'Mrs. Black.' Don't you remember she is married to Daddy's best friend from high school, Mark Green?"

Mary makes the occasional mistake with names, dates and places. Thanks to her sense of humor, she manages to cover up the mistakes by making a joke of it. She gets along well with homemaking, travel, volunteer work and socialization. Sometimes she worries

Global Deterioration Scale

Stage	Cognitive Decline	Characteristics
1	No decline	No notable memory problems
2	Very mild	Forgetful, socially appropriate
3	Mild	Early confusion; anxious, concentration difficult, denial
4	Moderate	Notable deficits, forgets recent events, problems with money and mobility, more concrete thinking
5	Moderate severe	Early dementia, simple assistance with activities of daily living, skill losses, some disorientation
6	Severe	Middle dementia, minimal memory access, possible incontinence, extreme emotional or behavioral changes, needs supervision for activities of daily living
7	Very severe	Late dementia, incontinence, lack of verbal communication, brain cannot control locomotion or respond to basic directions

Adapted from Reisberg, B., Ferris, S.H., et al. (1982). The global deterioration scale for assessment of primary degenerative dementia. *American Journal of Psychiatry*, 139, 1136-1139.

about forgetfulness, but she doesn't want to talk about it with her son and daughter-in-law.

LeTran: Stage 3   Mild Cognitive Decline

"A fellow can only do so much fishing, then he needs real work." LeTran wasn't ready for total retirement, so he took a part-time job delivering supplies for a local hardware store. His wife, Mai, agreed that LeTran was happier since taking the job. That's why she was surprised when LeTran exploded and shouted "stop quizzing me" just because she asked if he had a pleasant day at work. Meanwhile LeTran's coworkers are just as surprised. Initially they were impressed at how much he knew about hardware and home repairs.

Because LeTran is such a likable man, the clerks are covering up his mistakes in packing the orders. Twice last week, LeTran forgot to make deliveries to job sites for contractors that are regular customers. The problems all came to light after the manager found out that LeTran entered $10 in the cash register for a $110 drill set. Thinking the job too stressful, the manager asked LeTran to see a counselor. At first LeTran felt his honesty was in question. Then he became anxious and confused. Certain that counseling is only for "people who are losing their minds," LeTran quit his job. He sees this as a "great shame on his family name." So he's been hanging around the downtown park for several days rather than go home and tell Mai what really happened at the hardware store.

Vivien: Stage 4   Moderate Cognitive Decline

"I can't believe you would take that doctor's word over mine." Vivien continues to chastise her daughter, Adrienne, on the drive home from the University Geriatric Clinic. The gerontologist confirmed what Adrienne thought; Vivien shows definite signs of cognitive decline and confusion consistent with the early stages of memory impairment. Vivien denies memory problems as ardently as she denies backing her car into the fence gate (even though the neighbor saw it happen).

Adrienne still sees in her mother the stubbornness and independence that helped her move to the city as a young widow with a toddler. During her lifetime, Vivien has backpacked in Europe, sailed the Caribbean and gone on a photo safari in Africa. In the five years since retiring from the CPA firm she co-founded, she grows less able to manage plans and schedules. Last month, Vivien's checking account was overdrawn again and she wandered away from a tour group, causing the entire group to miss their airplane connection. At other times, Vivien recalls amazing details from her business and personal life. Adrienne wants to help but Vivien tries to hide her confusion by insisting, "I'm fine, my brain is just a little tired from too many years of figuring tax returns."

Tyronne: Stage 5   Moderately Severe Cognitive Decline

"But I have to wear my school jacket when I meet my boys for track practice", Tyronne insisted, clinging to the fleece-lined jacket that was totally unsuited to the 90 degree temperature outside the nursing home. Tyronne often retreats into memories of his years as a high school track and field coach. He can tell you the statistics on his best runners and those of his favorite athlete, Jesse Owens. But on his last weekend at home, he tried to "recruit those fine, tall athletes" who were actually his grandsons.

Tyronne talks about walking miles to school and working his way through college to fulfill a promise to his mother about getting a good education. During a recent evaluation, he forgot the days of the week and could not even begin to count backward from 20 by twos. His oldest son, T.J. (Tyronne, Jr.) used to bring his dad home for an occasional weekend visit until the obsessive outbursts began. Since Tyronne doesn't remember T.J.'s wife, Shandra or her Aunt Minnie, who lives there, he acts as if the women are intruders. "Get those women out of my locker room, now!" Tyronne shouts repeatedly. He can no longer understand who they are or how they fit into his increasingly limited awareness of the environment.

Elena: Stage 6   Severe Cognitive Decline

"You are not my Esteban! Go away and bring him back to me." Once again, Esteban tries not to show how hurt he feels to be rejected by Elena, his wife of 52 years. Maybe he was wrong to hope that she would stop being as confused and nervous in the nursing home as she had been when he tried to care for her at home. Some days when he arrives to have lunch with Elena, she is like her former cheerful self. They sing together the Spanish folk songs that they learned as children. He brings letters and pictures from their large extended family to remind her about the many people who love her.

Yesterday when the priest visited, Elena cursed at him and walked away talking to her "new sister Carmen" (an imaginary person). Later she screamed at her unsuspecting roommate for being "disloyal to our family traditions."

Esteban knew that dementia would cause increasing memory loss and changes in behavior. He never expected to see his gentle, gracious wife act rude, disrespectful and angry. Still he faithfully comes to the nursing home every day to help her with lunch and dinner. Everyday the Elena he loves slips further away, never to return again.

Cal: Stage 7   Very Severe Cognitive Decline

"Good morning, Cal. I am glad to see you." Cal can no longer put sounds together to make words to greet Joanne. He grunts and moans. He cannot connect words with thoughts and actions. His body won't respond to spoken requests. He is not able to turn or raise himself, not even to ease discomfort, so he must be turned periodically to prevent bedsores. His entire world has collapsed into the space surrounding his bed, even this limited space is far beyond his grasp. Cal is dependent on another human being to fulfill his every need.

Most of his friends stopped visiting because they are disturbed by his uncontrolled movements and odd noises. His wife, Bonnie, died several years ago. All the more reason that Cally, his daughter from out of state, is thankful for Joanne. "Joanne is more than a caregiver to my father. She is his lifeline to care with dignity."

Cal is totally dependent on the nursing home staff. He is incontinent, unable to sit without support and needs help with feeding. His language abilities are completely absent. Trying to give him choices of food or clothing gets no discernible response. Still Joanne approaches Cal with the same genuine attentiveness that helped her get past his confusion and resistance when he entered the nursing home after his wife's sudden death several years ago. She is able to see and relate to the person beyond the ravages of the disease. Cal's cognitive decline has been rapid. The psychomotor skill deficits and neurologic symptoms signal that Cal is trapped inside the final stage of dementia.

Neurological Symptoms of Memory Impairment

Neurological deficits in language, sensory perception and motor skills can be found among persons with both reversible and irreversible memory impairments. The three types of deficits are: *aphasia* (language), *agnosia* (sensory perception) and *apraxia* (motor skills).

Loss of language skills including the ability to read or write is called *aphasia*. In addition to those losses, a person with aphasia may also become unable to understand spoken or written words. These general characteristics are part of aphasia, however, the types and extent of losses are not the same in all persons. One resident may be unable to respond to verbal directions, yet comprehend the same directions given in written or pictorial form. Another resident may speak clear and distinct words, but the spoken words and meanings are not congruent.

Persons with aphasia experience tremendous frustration trying to express themselves without realizing the confusion transmitted in their messages. Cal's grunting and moaning are efforts to communicate. As he reached the late stage of dementia, his sounds are unrecognizable as words. In dealing with total communication deficit, caregivers learn to pay careful attention to nonverbal cues such as facial expressions or gestures in order to receive the real message.

Agnosia is a loss of the sensory perceptions necessary to identify a person, place or object. Like Elena, a person with agnosia may not recognize a spouse, family member, or regular caregiver. With agnosia comes fear of the "stranger" who is no longer known and anger at what seems a deception. In extreme cases, a person with agnosia fails to recognize his or her own image in a mirror.

A person with agnosia can lose a lifelong sense of depth perception, falling on a single step by not stepping up or down to meet the change of levels. Some residents lose the ability to navigate around their rooms without bumping into furniture. Others forget how to use familiar objects and are found brushing their hair with a toothbrush full of paste.

Decline in motor skills known as *apraxia* may begin gradually or suddenly with some conditions. Adults have a huge menu of motor skills that are taken for granted. Dialing the telephone, tying shoe laces, buttoning a shirt and using a soup spoon are motor skills learned long ago and repeated with almost no thought. A person with apraxia may begin one of those motor skill activities, then become confused or forget during the process. Tyronne becomes extremely upset with himself when he loses focus while getting dressed. He still has the body of an athlete, strong and muscular. Unfortunately as his level of apraxia increases, he becomes less capable of performing basic motor skill tasks.

In early stages of apraxia, a caregiver can prompt the resident by modeling the motor skill one easy step at a time. Persons with reversible dementia conditions are taught again to perform these tasks. In later stages of irreversible dementia, re-learning is not possible and modeling is increasingly less effective. The time may arrive when the resident's level of apraxia is so great that following the caregiver's prompt is not possible. At that point, the caregiver assumes a greater role in performing these tasks for the resident.

Behavioral and Psychological Symptoms of Memory Impairment

Persons with memory impairment forget many things, including the polite behaviors and self-control expected in a social setting. After a lifetime of conforming to the socially and culturally accepted behaviors, the sudden onset of odd actions give an early clue that something is wrong. Some behaviors are different or opposite those expected of an adult. The change is also confusing to the person who can't seem to moderate his or her actions anymore. Vivien refused to admit to her daughter or the gerontologist that anything was wrong. She tries to cover up her own distress at actions and responses that seem to "come out of nowhere."

Other behaviors are so erratic, so extreme or so disruptive as to clearly be "problem behaviors."

A problem behavior interrupts functioning in a way that endangers the safety of the individual or other persons in the environment.

Labeling an action a "problem behavior" is often based on each caregiver's perception of what constitutes a problem. One caregiver is easily distressed when a resident persists in trying to put feet into armholes of a sweater. A caregiver on a later shift has no such problem if the same resident is given more time and modeling in how to put on each garment. Other types of behaviors are more generally agreed upon as "problems" that demand an immediate and appropriate response by the caregiver.

Typical "Problem" Behaviors of Memory Impairment

Anger
Whether a slow burn or a flash fire, the memory impaired person cannot explain the cause of distress that exploded into the anger outburst.

Anxiety
Memory impaired persons are often described as "fidgeting, nervous and fearful." The confusion that envelopes their lives creates a kind of uncertainty that results in the anxious mood.

Clinging
The confused person seeks security by staying close to a familiar caregiver or family member. When the caregiver is out of sight, even momentarily in the next room, the memory impaired person may feel great fear of abandonment.

Cursing
Family members are often shocked when their very polite grandparent curses loudly in public places. The cursing is another attempt to express frustration even though it is "out of character" compared with a person's behavior prior to becoming memory impaired.

Combativeness
As with cursing, combativeness occurs even with persons who were never known to be physically violent or abusive toward others. Kicking, hitting, punching and biting are the more common forms of combativeness among the memory impaired.

Depressed mood
In the early stages of confusion and memory impairment, depressed mood marked by sadness and isolation is a serious problem. As a person realizes that his or her behaviors are odd and ability to function independently is decreasing, the risk of clinical depression is high.

Disturbed Sleep
To the memory impaired adult, days and nights are easily confused. Sleep cycles become disrupted and irregular. Many times an exhausted spouse has been awakened at three o'clock in the morning by her husband who insists that they are "late for an important appointment."

Hallucinations

A memory impaired person who is deeply affected by agnosia (loss of sensory perceptions) can become very disturbed by seeing, hearing, or feeling things that do not exist. Hallucinations of people, animals, or fearful events are terrifying to the confused and memory impaired who do not understand efforts to reassure them about their safety.

Hoarding Food or Objects

A person with memory impairment strives to hold onto the world by closely guarding food or objects. On a very basic level, food is comfort and satisfaction. Objects may be personal possessions or items that belong to others. The hoarder is not a thief and does not recall either the act of taking something or hiding it.

Incontinence

Although a memory impaired person can toilet with assistance, s/he may forget what needs to be done while on the way to the bathroom.

Paranoia

Inability to distinguish friends from enemies leaves some memory impaired persons to form faulty beliefs about caregivers and family members. Memory impaired persons typically fear being poisoned, held captive, cheated, or threatened. Without warning, those irrational fears are directed at caregivers, spouse and family members.

Repetitive Actions

In an effort to find comfort, a person with memory impairment repeats the same question (When is lunch?) or spends long periods of time folding and unfolding a blanket. Some actions are harmless. Other harmful actions such as picking at the skin need redirection for safety and well being of the impaired adult.

Screaming

Raised voices do get attention. If the screaming is not about danger or needs, then it is more likely an expression of frustration or fear. Screaming is never a deliberate attempt to irritate the caregiver. The memory impaired person is not capable of plotting and performing vengeful acts.

Sexual Inappropriateness

Taking off clothing, masturbating and trying to touch other persons are not defiant or aggressive actions for memory impaired persons. They do not remember social rules and taboos. Behaving like the flower children of the 1960's, "if it feels good, do it" best describes the sexual behaviors of the memory impaired.

Territorial Protectiveness

Trying to find a secure place, memory impaired persons guard their personal space even when that area is a common area. Pushing and shoving matches happen when one resident uses the chair that another resident believes is his property (whether it is or not).

3

Assessment of the Memory Impaired Adult

Recognize assessment issues that are important to memory impaired persons, their families and their caregivers.

Identify differences between formal assessment and informal assessment

Preparation, training and application of a basic assessment system

Recognizing the Need for Assessment

Several times Adrienne dialed the telephone number. Hearing the receptionist answer, "University Geriatric Clinic, may I help you?" she hung up the telephone. Even with all the odd things that happened, Adrienne can't think of her active, healthy mother, Vivien, as "senile." Then came several embarrassing events that she could not ignore.

The Golden Travelers tour group leader says that her mother is not welcome on the group's next trip. Vivien's wandering away from the airport terminal caused a police alert and resulted in extra costs to every group member for a later flight out of Paris. The tour leader asked the group to overlook other quirky things Vivien did on the last two trips, but this was the last straw.

Adrienne still cringes at the tense scene of last week when she questioned her mother about damage to the car fender and fence gate. After Adrienne left, Vivien became overwhelmed with a desire to prove that she did not hit the fence. In her mind, details became confused. The action Vivien took created even more problems. By the time Adrienne was paged and returned to the house, she found a shouting match in the front yard involving her mother, a police officer, the teenager who mows the yard, and his parents. Vivien had called the police to report that fifteen-year-old Greg "probably drove my car without permission and dented the fender the day he came over to mow the lawn." The commotion drew the attention of Ellen, the next door neighbor, who felt she could no longer "protect Vivien." She told the police officer that she saw Vivien back into the gate and keep going as if nothing happened. The police officer did a great job of defusing this tense situation. Before leaving, he asked if Vivien had memory problems. He told Adrienne about the difficulty his family had in recognizing his grandfather's memory impairment. He recommended that she get an appointment for Vivien at the University Geriatric Clinic.

On the drive to the clinic, Vivien refused to talk. Adrienne wondered which choice was worse; let her mother be arrested for disorderly conduct or take her for a dementia assessment. Both choices seemed unacceptable.

Importance of Building Rapport at First Contact

Adrienne looked around the sunny patio-like reception room for a magazine large enough to hide behind. Without a shred of her usual tact, Vivien pointed at various clients and said loudly, "You don't think I'm like those old people do you?" Adrienne wanted to blend into the wallpaper. This attractively dressed woman next to her looked like her mother, but she certainly didn't behave anything like her.

They were shown to an office and introduced to Dr. Craig Taylor, a staff gerontologist. His calm, easygoing manner helped Vivien and Adrienne to drop their defenses. He asked Vivien if, as a mother, there were times when she sensed something was not quite right with her child before the child was able to ask for help. When that occurred didn't she question and search until she found the problem? "Of course I did," Vivien answered with maternal pride. "Then you know something about the importance of an assessment," Dr. Taylor replied.

"Looks to me like the circle of love and care that you created as a parent is now being extended by Adrienne to help you."

As Adrienne returned to the reception room to await completion of the preliminary evaluation, she was so thankful. Dr. Taylor's explanations about the assessment process made it seem more personal and less clinical than she expected.

Dealing with Denial

The same Dr. Taylor who was a "fine young man" and "a kind person" quickly became a "smart-aleck quack" in Vivien's thinking. Her opinion changed after hearing his recommendation for further testing at the clinic's Memory Impairment Pavilion. Adrienne apologized for her mother's angry outburst and agreed to bring her back for another appointment. Dashing down the hall, she wondered how she could persuade Vivien to return to the clinic.

After an hour in downtown traffic under the drone of her mother's non-stop griping, Adrienne arrived home. She told her husband, Kyle, that she needed some time alone before discussing what happened at the clinic. Retreating to the bathroom to soak in a hot bath, Adrienne replayed the events. "Maybe mother is right, she's just trying to do too much and not getting enough rest. Mother is the sharpest lady I've ever known, could I be overreacting? Anyone can have a little fender-bender, after all, no one was hurt."

Denial is affecting both mother and daughter. Confusion and fear are behind Vivien's denial. Adrienne's denial is an effort to avoid admitting that her mother is vulnerable. Even her mother's irrational explanations are easier to accept than Dr. Taylor's conclusion that she appears to be in the early stages of memory impairment. Adrienne always thought that she would get a phone call from the State Department saying that her mother died climbing in the Himalayan Mountains. She never imagined that mother might lose her vibrant personality and life experiences to dementia. "No, this can't be happening, not to my mother."

How Is Memory Impairment Diagnosed?

The most common type of memory impairment, Alzheimer's disease, can be identified through assessment and some medical testing.

Although families are told that their loved one is "diagnosed" with Alzheimer's, a fine line of difference needs to be understood. By way of comparison, consider a person with the symptoms of diabetes. A physician orders medical tests that confirm the condition identified (or diagnosed) as diabetes. Once diagnosed, diabetes can be treated with a variety of options such as diet, exercise, and medication. The condition "diabetes" meets the "diagnostic criteria," or set of symptoms and measures of body functions that distinguish diabetes from wellness.

Alzheimer's and other types of memory impairment are far more difficult to identify. Based on current medical knowledge, Alzheimer's cannot be "diagnosed" with certainty in a living person. That's because the plaque and neurofibrillary tangles of nerve fibers found in the brain of a person with Alzheimer's disease can only be verified after death by autopsy. Sophisticated medical equipment such as positron emission tomography scan (PET), single photon emission computed tomography (SPECT), magnetic resonance imaging (MRI) and computerized tomography (CT) are promising alternatives used to view abnormalities of the brain in a living person. As exciting as these technological options are, high costs and limited availability restrict their uses. Generally, a "diagnosis" of Alzheimer's is made by clinical interview, medical examination, psychological testing and family history.

Think about the initial stage of the diagnostic process as shown in Vivien's first meeting with the gerontologist, Dr. Taylor. The process begins with an "assessment." The clinical interview, medical examination, psychological testing, and family history are typical elements of an assessment for memory impairment. What is learned from the assessment may result in a "diagnosis." Or the assessment may support a "rule-out diagnosis," where certain specific cognitive or behavioral mental problems are eliminated. The complexity of these diagnostic and assessment processes go far beyond the purposes of this text. Enough is accomplished in creating an awareness among family and caregivers of the difficulties and multi-faceted approaches that are used to "diagnose" or identify memory impairment.

Formal Assessment and Informal Assessment

Dr. Taylor tried to reduce the mystery of an assessment by comparing it to a mother's efforts to identify or eliminate possible causes of a child's discomfort. He was right in showing that an assessment is not just a complex process for professionals. Informal assessment is done by all of us daily in many aspects of our lives. For example, when the kitchen drain is clogged, the person at the sink begins an assessment of the problem and searches for possible causes. A specialist (plumber) is called to make a "diagnosis" of the problem and suggest treatment ("use drain cleaner monthly and don't pour grease down the sink"). In the plumbing example as with memory impairment, the family or friends discover the problem long before specialists are called in for a formal assessment. The point to remember from this example is that the informal assessment (interactions and observations) of family and friends are very important to the formal assessment for memory impairment.

Formal assessment for Vivien actually began with the basic information that was requested when Adrienne made the appointment. The University Geriatric Clinic associate asked basic questions about Vivien including: name, address, phone number, date of birth, social security number, name of referring physician, name of any current medications and a description of the behaviors or symptoms that cause concerns about memory impairment.

On the day of the first appointment at the clinic, Adrienne was given a more detailed form to complete about her mother's health, nutrition, medications, mental status, cognitive functioning, changes in behaviors and ability to manage activities of daily living. Although Adrienne is not a full-time caregiver, she has the closest relationship to her mother of any family member. Based on a lifetime of observing and interacting with Vivien, Adrienne's informal assessment identified problems in behaviors and memory that need further evaluation for her mother's safety and wellbeing.

Assessment Is A Mandate, Not An Option

For Vivien and other community dwelling elders, assessment for memory impairment does not usually happen until erratic behaviors or life management problems come to the attention of family, friends, neighbors or a physician. Older persons who live in assisted care or nursing homes are more likely to receive periodic assessments. Much credit for the revitalized emphasis on assessment goes to a major study in 1988 by National Institutes of Health (NIH). The NIH consensus report firmly stated that a link between geriatric assessment and care plans was vital in dealing with depression. In the years since that report, elder care facilities have received increased pressure from state and federal regulatory agencies to show a link between assessment and care for other issues besides depression.

Over the past twenty years, most elder care facilities have established procedures for some type of assessment prior to accepting the elder as a resident. Follow-up assessments occur as required by state law or proactively, as deemed necessary by the care plan team.

For example, Tyronne is a resident at an assisted living center that conducts complete follow-up assessments twice annually with evaluations at each care plan team meeting. The staff social worker has worked with Tyronne on both assessments since he was admitted to the facility a year ago. His behaviors were still subject to angry outbursts and confusion, however, his cognitive skills were near to levels recorded at intake. A noticeable decline in cognitive skills (counting backward from 20 by twos) and reality orientation (did not know present day, date, or season) was discovered at the bi-annual assessment this month.

Tyronne's son, T.J., appreciates how carefully the care plan team responds to needs identified in the assessment. That's what he looked for when he made the tough decision to move his father from City Nursing Center closer to his home to We Care Village across town. At City Nursing Center, T.J. never felt confident that the staff had any coordinated care concept for each resident. He realized that his instincts were right after visiting We Care Village. During the eighteen months that Tyronne has lived at We Care Village, he is noticeably more alert and involved in activities. *The Caring Hearts Newsletter* and Our Families Care Support Group are still more responses to the requests by families of residents to be better informed. As a family member who needs reassurance about his father's safety, comfort and motivation to use remaining skills, T.J. has learned the difference between a facility that really uses assessments to help residents and one that merely goes through the motions.

Attitudes Toward Assessment

Assessment, implemented as a requirement without solid follow-up care and monitoring, may fulfill the letter of the law, but certainly not the intent. That's the traditional caretaking approach. Why does a facility take a negative attitude toward assessment? There are four basic reasons:

1. time constraints
2. focus on assessment as a requirement rather than a benefit
3. inadequate staff training in assessment
4. minimal assessment is consistent with a less individualized approach to care

The opposite is true for enlightened caregiving, like T.J. found at We Care Village. This facility places great value on assessment in developing a comprehensive care plan for every resident. Development of a comprehensive care plan relies on formal assessment (i.e., cognitive testing, skills evaluation, medical testing) and informal assessment (i.e., observations from family, caregivers, and support staff). The input of everyone who interacts with a resident on a regular basis is important. Once the assessment is complete with goals defined, the comprehensive care plan approach is shared with all departments of the facility to enlist everyone's participation.

A Family Perspective on Assessment

Families encountering memory impaired problems for the first time typically respond like Adrienne with a mixture of uncertainty, relief and denial. The questions that lead to an assessment appointment sound like the following. *Something needs to be done, but what? How serious is the problem? Is it temporary? What do we need to do next? Is home care possible or must we find a nursing home?*

An effective assessment answers some, but not all the questions that families have about memory impairment.

Although this chapter gives direction to facility staff and those who conduct assessments, it's also important to families. Understanding the "insider information" about the overall purpose and approach to the assessment helps families to realize that nothing strange or demeaning will happen to their loved ones. An assessment is merely a measurement of skills and functioning to be used in treatment planning or in directing family caregivers how to best work with the memory impaired resident.

A Working Assessment System

First and foremost, a working assessment system is one that works for the resident and is workable for the staff. A workable assessment system is:

> Multi-Modal
> Flexible
> Sensitive
> Reliable
> User-Friendly

Multi-Modal approach to mental health is based on Arnold Lazarus' (1976) approach to evaluation, the BASIC ID. Using that acronym as a guide for assessment of a memory impaired person directs attention to these areas:

> Behavior - actions, reactions
> Affect - mood, feelings, emotions
> Sensation - sensory input and responses
> Imagery - abstraction, forming mental pictures
> Cognition - active thinking and memory
> Interpersonal Relationships - socialization
> Diet or Drugs - influences of these elements on physical
>   and emotional well-being

The *multi-modal* approach seeks a wide range of information about a person from physical, mental, emotional, relational and behavioral perspectives. Compare the new information at each assessment with that obtained at the intake assessment and a richer picture of the resident's abilities and needs emerges.

A workable assessment system needs to be flexible enough to be useful with residents at various levels of impairment. Prepare in advance a compact package of materials for the assessment. The most useful assessments may be done "on the move." The person conducting the assessment may be called to a home, adult day care center or retirement community. The resident being assessed may be more verbal while walking and talking than seated in a traditional assessment setting. At the very least, walking with the resident can build rapport prior to testing that needs to be done while seated and using special materials.

Even inside a nursing home, the location of the assessment can vary. In this author's experience, restless memory impaired residents can sometimes focus better when the assessment is conducted in their rooms, in a sitting room, or outdoors at a picnic table on the unit's patio. Staying flexible enough to find a location in which the resident feels at ease is worth the effort. Forget the white lab coats and dull testing rooms. Many basic assessment tools are easily portable. Prepare to be pleasantly surprised at how much more is accomplished with those memory impaired residents who respond poorly to traditional testing room set-ups.

For an assessment to be useful over time, it must be sensitive to changes in the cognitive skills and functioning levels of memory impaired persons. It is equally important to find assessment tools that are culturally sensitive. An effective assessment helps the care planning team determine if recent behavioral changes are pervasive or situational. Answering that question is significant in making adjustments to care plans or medication evaluations.

Reliable results are imperative in making care plans for the memory impaired. In order to be used for determining mental status or psychological functioning, an assessment instrument must be valid and reliable. These terms are taken from statistics. A valid assessment is one that measures what it is intended to measure. For example, a test that measures depression would not give adequate information about cognitive functioning. A memory impaired person may have significant cognitive losses without displaying depressed symptoms. Thus a test for depression would not be a valid measure of cognitive functioning in this example.

To be reliable, a test must have a high degree of accuracy in measuring what it is designed to measure. Some tests have two parts that allow for a test and a retest. If a person is given a reliable test in two parts by different administrators, then the results will be similar. More complex issues exist in test design, however, these issues go beyond what is needed for this text. Simply remember that a reliable assessment instrument gives information that can be relied upon to assist in care planning.

User-friendly is a term not always connected with assessment. Many psychological and neuropsychological assessments require master's or doctoral training to perform. Don't be turned off to assessment tools because of the some complex types. Plenty of practical assessment instruments are available that are user-friendly and more useful for day-to-day care plan needs of the memory impaired. A user-friendly assessment system is cost efficient, transportable, and suitable for administration by several members of the regular staff. Please remember this critical caution: a caregiver needs training and supervision as appropriate to the assessment instrument. Without proper administration and scoring, the results obtained are useless. In a worst case situation, inaccurate results could bring about care plan decisions that are harmful to the memory impaired resident.

Another aspect of a user-friendly assessment is that it provides information to assist caregivers at every level in working with a memory impaired resident. An assessment that only the staff psychologist can understand offers no help to the occupational therapist or the dietary aide who works regularly with the resident. Information from the assessment must be communicated in language that everyone on the care plan team can understand.

Preparing to Conduct an Assessment

The care plan team, physician, or individual caregiver may decide that an assessment is needed and make the appropriate request. In making plans for an assessment, the seven important factors to consider are: purpose, problems, prerequisites, physical, psychological, personal, and prescription.

Determining the purpose for an assessment is the first step.
Begin by asking "why?" Why is the assessment needed? Why is it needed now? Poor answers such as "because the psychologist is available today" or "the family wants more information" are not acceptable reasons for scheduling an assessment. The better question is, "can this resident benefit from information obtained in

this assessment at this time?" If the answer is yes, then proceed to clarify the resident's status on the other factors.

Assessments are helpful in identifying problems.

As an example, consider an older person whose erratic outbursts frighten family members and cause embarrassing scenes in public. A physical examination fails to show any medical reasons for the unusual behaviors. A basic assessment of cognitive processing gives the initial clue that memory impairment is suspected. Later a neuro-psychological assessment identifies visual-spatial disorientation and motor disturbances in walking (gait) that is consistent with dementia symptoms noted in the basic assessment.

Even after the initial diagnosis of dementia is made, assessments are still useful to identify a person's remaining strengths and challenges. A periodic repeat of basic cognitive functioning assessment gives useful information to the care plan team on the level of skill decline or maintenance since the last measurement. Specific problems may also be assessed such as measurement of depressive symptoms.

The prerequisites to a well planned assessment include reviewing the social history, intake recommendations, prior assessment reports, and comments or requests from family members.

In assessments there is no such thing as too much information. The clues of how to connect with each resident are waiting discovery. Like a skilled detective, the assessor and care plan team become as familiar as possible with each resident prior to assessment.

Obtain a recent evaluation from the physician to determine how much, if at all, physical (medical) conditions are part of the overall problems.

Physical conditions such as hypoglycemia, hypothyroidism, and vitamin B-12 deficiencies are just a few potential causes of dementia due to general medical conditions. Add these medical complications to an existing memory impairment and the already declining condition grows dramatically more severe. Bringing relief to a medical complication may be what is needed to ease the psychological and cognitive stresses. The choice may be to go no further in the assessment process until the medical complications are managed.

Psychological distress accounts for the most disruptive types of behavioral symptoms.
If the emotional impact of disruptive behaviors is tough on family and caregivers, realize that it's even more disturbing to the confused, memory impaired person. For some persons, the psychological symptoms measured in the assessment are transient, such as fear, anxiety, anger, or combativeness. Other symptoms are pervasive indicating deeper levels of distress such as hallucinations, delusions, paranoia, or depression. If psychological symptoms are prominent in the basic assessment, another more sophisticated psychological or neuropsychological assessment with a qualified assessor is desirable.

Personal satisfaction and quality of life are sought by all persons, including the memory impaired.
Any type of assessment needs to pay attention to the personal concerns. A memory impaired person may be more expressive nonverbally if verbal communication is too confusing. During all phases of the assessment, the assessor must remain aware of any and all ways that a memory impaired person is trying to communicate.

The caregivers must be willing and able to work with the prescription or the recommendations that emerge from the assessment.
The most comprehensive assessment conducted by the highest ranking specialist in memory impairment is just so much wasted paper unless the recommendations are put into action. A well written assessment report is expected to have goals that are "operationalized" or stated in action-oriented terms. Specific suggestions of what to do or not to do also need to be clarified. Otherwise, an assessment report filled with charts and numbers is not useful in day-to-day caregiving. Finally, the actions recommended in the assessment need to be integrated into the overall care plan and monitored.

Practical Guidelines for Conducting the Assessment

Whoever is chosen to handle the formal assessment of a memory impaired person benefits from following five guidelines to create a climate of ease and comfort during the process.

Remember, these guidelines are directed to facility staff members who have qualifications appropriate to conduct assessments.

Practice or review the assessment instruments before using with a resident.

Ask a co-worker to play the role of resident while you conduct the assessment. An experienced assessor may need only to re-read the instruments and administration directions to be prepared for working with residents. Both experienced and novice assessors benefit from observing an assessment done by another staff member.

Identify several potential locations for the assessment.

Every effort must be made to preserve the integrity of the assessment. With some instruments, that means total privacy to avoid any other input. However, assessment of memory impaired persons requires more flexibility. As previously mentioned, a restless resident who can't sit still or gets nervous in a closed room, may actually give more focus to the assessment in non-traditional areas.

Prior to the assessment, the assessor needs to identify at least three possible locations. For example, in a certain facility the three locations might be a quiet office or sitting room, the resident's room, or in rocking chairs on the patio. The patio may be less "private" in that other people could walk around the area, and yet be more comfortable for the resident. Certainly interference by other residents with the assessment means that the assessor stops and begins again at a later time or the next day.

Collect all supplies before beginning.

Memory impaired residents are easily distracted and sometimes very impatient. Don't expect these residents to "wait right here while I sharpen another pencil." Leave the room, answer a phone call or otherwise break the continuity of the assessment, and the resident may not be able to get back on task.

Bring extra supplies for each assessment. If the resident is asked to write or draw, have several sizes of pens, pencils or large markers. Persons with arthritis in their hands often find the larger markers or pencils easier to use. If there is no table, a lap board or large clip board may give stability to paperwork for both assessor and resident.

Whatever is needed for the assessment, bring plenty of materials and have it ready to use before going to find the resident.

Set a comfortable pace.

The assessor can match the resident's pace or set a more moderate pace as needed to interact with a fidgety resident. Keep it conversational, not monotone. If appropriate to the instrument, allow the resident some time to explain answers. The act of listening is a sign of respect that is as important to the memory impaired as to anyone. The assessor's desire to complete the instrument does not justify rushing the resident to answer. If there is not enough time to administer the assessment at a comfortable, conversational pace, then re-schedule for another time.

Avoid creating a distraction when recording responses.

Some assessors become so busy reading the questions and recording the answers that they barely make eye contact with the person being assessed. The pre-occupation with writing and shuffling answer sheets is distracting to anyone. To a memory impaired person, that much distraction is enough to ruin the assessment.

This problem can be managed in two ways. First, practice with a co-worker or read the assessment questions aloud several times while looking in the mirror. Second, see how smoothly you can make notes on the test form while maintaining eye contact with yourself (and smiling) in a mirror. If practicing with a co-worker, ask that person to say "look up" anytime your focus lingers on the paper instead of the person. Above all, don't be discouraged. Many experienced assessment specialists recall that developing the skill to record responses unobtrusively was the most difficult aspect of learning to conduct assessments.

The extent to which the factors are managed and the guidelines are met, results in an assessment that is a satisfactory experience for both resident and assessor.

4

A Basic Assessment System

Overcoming communication problems

Examples of instruments that may be used for a Basic Assessment System

Preparing a Behavior Checklist that is useful for family and facility caregivers

A Basic Assessment System in Action

Preparing the assessment instruments and training the assessors is just like setting in place all the scenery, props and costumes before the play begins. How effectively the actors use the props and how well the scenery blends is not known until it is time for the performance. Getting ready for assessments is similar. All the advance work in preparing each element and supervising the assessors rehearsal with colleagues is done to make the actual assessment seem casual and comfortable for the person being assessed. As stated in the previous chapter, a look inside the assessment process helps new care providers learn how to assess or assist the assessor. Families discover that the assessment process is not mysterious, but useful and respectful. The following is an example of an assessment outreach.

"Before we leave for the Senior Center, let's review our materials and assignments," said Margaret Allen, social services director of University Geriatric Clinic. Two days each month this community outreach team visits senior adult programs around the county to conduct depression screenings and memory impairment assessments. Margaret, a licensed clinical social worker, leads this team of two nurses, two social work interns, and three intake specialists.

Today's location is the downtown Senior Center, visited quarterly by the clinic's outreach team. When the team arrives, the Senior Center's activities director points to a reception room filled with people who came for the assessment. The well-organized team gets right to work.

The first name on the list is LeTran. He and his wife, Mai, arrived very early even though he doesn't think he needs to be here. He's doing this to please Mai because she gets so upset when he forgets to do things. Last week, she showed him the flyer about the assessment. With tears in her eyes, Mai begged him to go to the assessment. So LeTran agreed to the assessment to satisfy Mai. And frankly, he hopes to disprove her ridiculous idea about memory problems by passing this assessment with flying colors.

When his name is called, LeTran and Mai are greeted by Tara Cartland, intake specialist. Tara explains her role in gathering background information about LeTran that will be useful for the assessment. Mai is asked to add any information that she thinks is important.

LeTran answers questions about his physical health and overall good condition. He doesn't take any prescription medications and walks regularly for exercise. His appetite is good. But then, he adds, "Mai is a wonderful cook." LeTran is becoming more confident about the questions. According to LeTran, his behaviors are the same as always. Tara asks Mai if that is what she observes. Mai tells about LeTran's more frequent angry outbursts, his frustration with simple household tasks and his forgetfulness. "How often do these behaviors occur," asks Tara. "Maybe a couple of times a year," says LeTran. "More like three or four times weekly," Mai corrects.

Tara's questions now focus on what she calls "activities of daily living, such as showering, dressing, feeding, and self management." LeTran replies that he is "totally capable of taking care of myself." Mai thinks about this morning when LeTran turned on the water in the shower and walked away. She reminded him to take a shower. Then he nearly left the house with mis-matched clothing. "He never used to be like this," Mai thought but did not want to say aloud. After finishing the intake forms, Tara escorts LeTran to a nearby office and Mai to the reception area.

As LeTran enters the testing room, Mark Bradley introduces himself as a social work intern with University Geriatric Clinic. He says that in addition to his interest in working with senior adults, he also likes fishing and reading. For a few minutes, Mark and LeTran talk about fishing. Even with a busy schedule of assessments, Mark was trained to take some time to build rapport that creates a conversational tone for the remainder of the interview.

Beginning with what Mark calls "school type questions," LeTran starts off confident then gets frustrated. He stumbles over the name of the current U.S. president and does not accurately name the previous president. When asked what is his mother's maiden name, his facial expression is confused as he takes several minutes to give an answer. As for the mental computation of subtracting three from 20 and continuing to subtract three from each number down, LeTran misses the first subtraction and is fidgety. While he goes to the restroom, Mark glances at the telephone number on the intake form: 512-3345. When asked to state his phone number, LeTran hesitated then replied: "512-334." He insisted that was accurate, even though he did not give enough digits for a complete phone number.

After LeTran returns, Mark asks him to answer "yes or no" to a series of thirty questions. LeTran responds quickly to some questions and takes longer with others. When asked if he has difficulty concentrating, making decisions, and getting upset over little things, LeTran answers "yes," then gives some confusing and contradictory explanations about those answers.

Based on the answers given, Mark notes that there is no evidence of depression but scores do indicate a problem with cognitive functioning. When the person being assessed scores in the range of mild to moderate cognitive impairment, the team's procedure is to use a second mental status test to affirm or challenge that result. From the beginning of the second test, LeTran becomes visibly anxious when he seems unsure of the answer. He complains that it's "stupid to spell a word backwards." On another question, Mark notes that LeTran must be guessing because he failed to recall the names of any of the three common objects (pen, notepad, stapler) that he identified a few minutes earlier.

The final task is for LeTran to draw interlocking geometric figures like those shown on a card Mark is holding. LeTran claims this is easy because he likes to draw and did well in commercial drafting class. He proudly hands his finished copy of the design to Mark. The lines are wavy and the angles do not accurately intersect as shown on the sample card.

When the testing is finished, Mark leaves briefly to consult with the team leader, Margaret. At LeTran's request, Mai is invited to join them to hear the results of the assessment. Mark reminds them that this is a basic assessment designed to indicate if further evaluation is needed. Margaret explains that as team leader and a licensed clinical social worker, she is here to explain what was discovered in the assessment. In a calm voice, Margaret reports; "LeTran does not show symptoms of depression, however, there are reasons to be concerned about mild levels of cognitive impairment or memory loss." LeTran casts an angry look at Mai and leaves the office saying he will "wait in the car."

Mai asks what she can do to help her husband. Margaret gives her a package of information that includes a list of local memory impairment support groups, a chart of the stages of memory impairment, a list of books written for families of the memory impaired and a description of follow-up services available at the University Geriatric Clinic. She directs Mai's attention to a prestamped fold-over reply card. "After thirty days, please note on this card any actions you decide to take, any new behavioral problems and whether you want to make an evaluation appointment at the clinic. Or, check the box indicating no further action desired. Your response helps us determine if we are adequately serving families with these outreach programs."

Mai clutches the package, wipes away a tear and forces a smile as she walks toward the car. She's thankful that LeTran is in the passenger seat and allowing her to drive home. Driving keeps her focused. He talks about fishing and she drives. Both are trying to adjust to the life-changing news that is so hard to accept.

The experience of LeTran and Mai shows how an assessment can confirm a family's worst fears. In other cases, an assessment may show that the real problems are much less severe than anticipated. Whatever the results, an assessment is the first step to dealing with reality in a constructive way.

Health care providers from physicians to nurses to social workers to patient care aides need to recognize the emotional impact on the spouse and family that happens following the discovery of memory impairment problems. Home health workers, adult daycare aides and physician's office assistants are often the most accessible people with whom families can talk about their concerns. Knowing all the answers isn't necessary. The best way to be helpful is to listen, acknowledge the concerns, and encourage families to contact a local memory impairment support group or nearby chapter of the Alzheimer's Association.

Preparing to Conduct the Assessment

The concept of an assessment system is familiar to some caregivers and a total mystery to others. Gaining more information about a memory impaired resident's cognitive functioning, moods, and behavioral symptoms makes it possible for caregivers at all levels to better identify and meet needs.

Methods of assessment vary according to what is measured and the expertise of the assessor. For example, complex neuropsychological assessments must be given and interpreted by a qualified psychologist. A much simpler test of mental status such as the *Short Portable Mental Status Questionnaire* (Pfeiffer, 1974) can be given and scored by persons with training in social work, nursing, and intake counseling. Both complex and simple tests yield useful information for care planning.

Keep in mind the key question about assessment from Chapter 5: "can this resident benefit from information obtained in this assessment at this time?" For some memory impaired residents, a full psychological or psychiatric assessment battery is needed, yet for other residents this approach would be excessive. Care plan teams are primarily interested in the practical needs of residents which are often effectively identified by simple assessments repeated at regular intervals. Simple can be better if the results obtained are useful in day to day care.

The *basic assessment system* presented in this text is suitable for administration by nurses, counselors, social workers and intake specialists. The information obtained from the basic assessment system is immediately useful for any care plan method.

Overcoming Communication Problems

Starting the assessment with a casual, conversational tone is important for making the respondent feel at ease. A respondent who feels safe and comfortable is more likely to cooperate with the assessor. The assessor sets the tone for the interview by greeting the respondent by name. "Good morning, Mary, my name is Jane. Please join me." Depending on the resident's mobility, the assessor makes a gesture toward the chair, offers an arm for support or assists in directing the wheelchair to the testing area. Begin with a few questions about personal comfort.

"Am I speaking so that you can hear me?"

If the respondent answers "yes," proceed with testing. If the respondent answers "no", ask the following questions while raising or lowering the voice volume.

"If I speak louder (increase volume), can you hear me now?"

"If I speak softer (lower volume), can you hear me now?"

For respondents who are wearing hearing devices, point toward the device and ask:

"Does your hearing aid need adjusting?"

Working with a respondent who indicates hearing problems (with or without a hearing device), suggest the following:

"Can you hear me better if I talk toward your left ear?"

"Can you hear me better if I talk toward your right ear?"

Some respondents are hesitant to tell you about any hearing problems. Asking these "personal comfort" questions helps the assessor to know at what point the respondent can hear adequately to complete the assessment. Terrible injustices have occurred when an unskilled assessor judged a person mentally incompetent who was actually hearing impaired. The inability to clearly hear and understand the full question prompted the incorrect answer.

The next step is to give reassurance about the purpose of the assessment.

"I wonder if you know the reason for this assessment?"

Allow time to answer. Listen carefully for the concerns expressed.

"I want to assure you that this assessment is to help me get to know you better. What I learn about you will be used by your care team (or family) to help you in everyday living."

Let's say that as the assessor, you have completed the "personal comfort" questions. A few other communication problems may arise such as the following:

The suspicious respondent feels like he or she is on trial and the assessor is the chief prosecutor. This respondent reluctantly gives "yes" or "no" answers, then pauses to watch the assessor's reactions. The assessor needs to give the respondent time to warm up to the process. Encourage the respondent to expand on an answer by saying, "I'd like to hear more about that" or "can you give me an example." After these efforts, if the respondent does not participate more freely, then accept the limited information given. The assessor makes a note about attempts to establish rapport and the respondent's continued reluctance.

The chatty respondent establishes rapport quickly then moves to take control of the assessment. This respondent may be lonely and looking for someone to listen. Or this respondent may be a person who drifts off into long stories as a way to dodge a direct question. The assessor need not be afraid to limit and redirect conversation back to the assessment. Use gentle redirection such as, "I'd enjoy hearing more about that later, now I need to ask you about…." Only use this redirection if you plan to allow a few minutes at the end of the assessment to let the respondent speak freely. Introduce that option at the end by saying, "in the five minutes we have left together, do you have anything more you need to tell me?"

To simply redirect a chatty respondent back to the question wait for a pause then comment, "let's return to the question about sleeping habits (or whatever the essence of the question)…." Another transition technique is to repeat the respondent's words, "I hear what you are saying about feeling blue, now let's talk about …."

The anxious respondent can be fearful or tearful. As with the suspicious respondent, the anxious respondent needs for the assessor to give repeated reassurance and patience. The tearful respondent benefits from a brief break in the assessment to regain composure. Offer a cup of water, a tissue or extend your hand for the respondent to hold.

The angry respondent is a real challenge to even an experienced assessor. Acknowledge the anger without focusing on it. "I understand you are angry about selling your home to move to the retirement center, now I need to get to know about other things that are important to you ... (return to next assessment question)." If the respondent directs anger at you, as the assessor, avoid getting drawn into a defensive position. Arguing about the value of the assessment, techniques or instruments is a losing game. When a respondent becomes verbally abusive or combative, discontinue the assessment.

The speech impaired respondent can complete the same assessment package if the assessor finds alternative ways for the person to answer. Rather than frustrate the respondent by not being able to understand him or her, have the solution ready in your testing materials. Here's how to prepare answer cards. Take three white, unlined 4×6 index cards. In bold black marker, print the words "YES", "NO," and "NOT SURE" on separate cards. Glue or tape each card to a tongue depressor. These three signs can be given to a speech impaired respondent to use for answering some assessment questions. Demonstrate by reading a sample question and holding up a sign as the answer.

Open-ended questions that require a respondent to give an opinion or recall information may be completed by using a marker board and bold markers. Allow the respondent ample time to write an answer. If none of these techniques work, assessment of the speech impaired respondent likely requires more specialized types of testing by either a speech therapist or psychologist.

The respondent who needs an interpreter is generally identified prior to the assessment. However, with community dwelling elders coming into a central assessment site (as in the story of LeTran), the assessor does not have advance notice. Whether the respondent needs an American Sign Language interpreter or a native language interpreter, the assessment cannot proceed until communication through a skilled interpreter is arranged. An assessor who learned conversational Spanish for travel or a volunteer who speaks a minimum of German lacks sufficient skills to be a qualified interpreter for assessments.

A Reminder for Novice and Experienced Assessors

Assessment of mental status, depression, or emotional adjustment is never as clear as seeing a broken bone on an x-ray. Cognitive and emotional problems are more difficult to identify and treat than some medical conditions. Never begin an assessment with an assumption about the findings. Trying to prove a preconceived notion usually results in slanting the assessment to prove a point rather than discover the respondents real needs.

Assessments require paperwork. Find a way to manage the papers (i.e., clipboard, folder, or side table) so that juggling papers does not become a distraction to the respondent. Another frequent distration for respondents is watching the assessor record answers on the scoring sheet. Record answers as unobstrusively as possible. Some respondents become very anxious or fearful that the assessor is "checking up on them" or "writing bad things." Accuracy without distracting movements is important.

Finally, the key to a good assessment is in the assessor's approach as summarized by the three B's: be familiar with the tests, be reassuring to the respondent, and be positive throughout the process from greeting to completion.

Instruments in a Basic Assessment System
Short Portable Mental Status Questionnaire
Mini-Mental State Exam
Geriatric Depression Scale
Behavior Checklist

These assessment instruments can be used separately or combined for a broader view of the resident's skills, mood, cognitive abilities and needs. Following the instruments is a useful form:
Assessment Summary Report

Guidelines for Administering the Short Portable Mental Status Questionnaire

1. Make an effort to ask every question.
2. Record every answer as stated by the respondent. All items in a question must be answered to give credit for that question.
3. If the respondent makes five (5) consecutive errors, stop the assessment. Thank the respondent for his/her answers. Do not indicate that the test was incomplete.
4. If the respondent has less than a high school education, the score is modified by subtracting one from the error score.
5. The assessor may repeat the question or encourage the respondent to answer. For example, if the respondent pauses in calculating the serial subtraction (#10), the assessor may say "and now, what is three from that number?" The assessor may not repeat the last number calculated by the respondent.

Scoring Key for Short Portable Mental Status Questionaire (SPMSQ)

Match the total number of respondent errors with the score in the following table. Note the "significance" of each numerical score. If the assessor is using a summary sheet, record the number of errors and the significance.

Score	Significance
0 - 2 Errors	Intellectually Intact
3 - 4 Errors	Mild Cognitive Impairment
5 - 7 Errors	Moderate Cognitive Impairment
8 - 10 Errors	Severe Cognitive Impairment

Short Portable Mental Status Questionnaire (SPMSQ)

Respondent name _____

Assessor name _____ Date _____

Assessor begins:
"I am going to ask you a few school type questions. How far did you go in school?"   _____ years or _____ grade.

Ask questions 1 - 10. Enter a "1" in column for correct or error.
Respondent may not refer to a newspaper, calendar or other aides.

Question	Correct	Error
1. What day is it? Month ___ Day ___ Year ___	___	___
2. What day of the week is it? _____	___	___
3. What is the name of this place? _____	___	___
4. What is your telephone number? _____	___	___
5. How old are you? Age _____	___	___
6. When were you born? Month _____ Day _____ Year _____	___	___
7. Who is the President of the United States now? _____	___	___
8. Who was President before him? _____	___	___
9. What is your Mother's maiden name? _____	___	___
10. Subtract 3 from 20 and keep subtracting 3 from each number all the way down. Entire series must be correct. _____	___	___

Total number of errors ___

Guidelines for Administering the Mini-Mental Status Exam

1. Make an effort to complete all questions.
2. Prior to testing prepare the following:
   using plain white paper withno lines, print in bold block letters this phrase: CLOSE YOUR EYES
3. Decide which three objects will be used for review and recall (Questions 3 & 5).
4. Have a pencil or marker for the respondent to use in copying the drawing.

Folstein, M.F., Folstein, S.E., & McHugh, P.R. (1975). Mini-mental state: a practical method for grading the cognitive state of patients for the clinician. *Journal of Psychiatric Research*, 12, 189-198. Used with permission. © 1975, Pergamon Journals Ltd.

Mini-Mental State Exam (MMSE)

Respondent: _____

Date _____ Score _____ (max = 30)

Orientation (1 point each correct)

1. What is the Day _____ Year _____ Season _____
   Date _____ Month _____

2. Where are we State _____ County _____ Town/
   City _____ Place/Dwelling _____ Floor _____

Registration (3 points)

3. Name three objects, taking one second to say each. Then ask patient all three after you have said them. Give 1 point for each correct answer. Repeat answers until patient learns all. _____

Attention and Calculation (5 points)

4. Serial sevens. Start with 7, add 7, then continue adding 7 to the next number four more times.1 point for each correct answer. Stop after five. OR Spell WORLD backwards. _____

Recall (3 points)

5. Ask for names of three objects learned in #3.
   1 point for each correct answer. _____

Language (see points after each question)

6. Point to a pencil and a watch. Have patient name them as you point. _____ (2)

7. Have patient repeat "No ifs, and, or buts" ___ (1)

8. Have patient follow three stage command; "Take the paper in your right hand, fold paper in half, hand paper to me " ___(3)

9. Have patient read and obey following: CLOSE YOUR EYES (written large letters) _____ (1)

10. Have patient write sentence of own choice. Must contain subject, object and make sense. Ignore spelling errors. ___ (1)

11. Have patient copy design on attached page.

    (1 point if all sides & angles preserved and intersecting sides form a quadrangle.) ___ (1)

Respondent: _____ Date _____

MMSE p. 2

Draw a copy of this design in the space below.

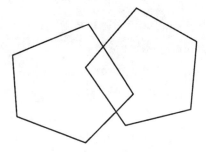

Guidelines for Administering Geriatric Depression Scale (GDS)

1. Read each question slowly and distinctly.
2. Ask respondent to say "Yes" or "No" as to how he/she feels about each question.
3. Introduce GDS as "a measure of how the respondent feels in different settings." Don't say "this is a depression inventory."

Yesavage, J.A, & Brink. T.L, (1983). *Development and validation of a Geriatric Depression Screening Scale.* Journal of Psychiatric Research, 17, 41. Used with permission. © 1983, Pergamon Journals Ltd.

Geriatric Depression Scale (GDS)

Respondent Name _____

Date_____   Score_____

Please answer each question by drawing a circle around either Y(Yes) or N (No)

Y N   1.   Are you basically satisfied with your life?

Y N   2.   Have you dropped many of your activities and interests?

Y N   3.   Do you feel that your life is empty?

Y N   4.   Do you often get bored?

Y N   5.   Are you hopeful about the future?

Y N   6.   Are you bothered by thoughts that you just can't get out of your head?

Y N   7.   Are you in good spirits most of the time?

Y N   8.   Are you afraid that something bad is going to happen to you?

Y N   9.   Do you feel happy most of the time?

Y N 10.   Do you often feel helpless?

Y N 11.   Do you often get restless and fidgety?

Y N 12.   Do you prefer to stay in home, rather than attend activities outside?

Y N 13.   Do you frequently worry about the future?

Y N 14. Do you feel that you have more problems with memory than most?

Y N 15. Do you think it is wonderful to be alive now?

Y N 16. Do you often feel downhearted and blue?

Y N 17. Do you feel pretty worthless the way you are now?

Y N 18. Do you worry a lot about the past?

Y N 19. Do you find life very exciting?

Y N 20. Is it hard to get started on new projects?

Y N 21. Do you feel full of energy?

Y N 22. Do you feel that your situation is hopeless?

Y N 23. Do you think that most people are better off than you?

Y N 24. Do you frequently get upset over little things?

Y N 25. Do you feel like crying?

Y N 26. Do you have trouble concentrating?

Y N 27. Do you enjoy getting up in the morning?

Y N 28. Do you prefer to avoid social gatherings?

Y N 29. Is it easy for you to make decisions?

Y N 30. Is your mind as clear as it used to be?

Scoring Key for Geriatric Depression Scale

The following are the "depressive responses." Each counts one point.

1.	N	11.	Y	21.	N
2.	Y	12.	Y	22.	Y
3.	Y	13.	Y	23.	Y
4.	Y	14.	Y	24.	Y
5.	N	15.	N	25.	Y
6.	Y	16.	Y	26.	Y
7.	N	17.	Y	27.	N
8.	Y	18.	Y	28.	Y
9.	N	19.	N	29.	N
10.	Y	20.	Y	30.	N

If the total number of depressive responses is:

    10 or less   normal

    11 - 20   mild depression

    21 - 30   moderate to severe depression

Guidelines for using Behavior Checklist

1. Prepared by a staff observer or home caregiver
2. Unlike other tests, there is no stated meaning to "scores." Rather, the scores are used to compare response changes over time.
3. Observations may be made alternate days over an eight day period. Another option is to make observations during day and evening hours. For facility caregivers, this will involve observation notes made on two shifts for several days.
4. Refer to Chapters two and seven for more information on the behaviors that are being rated on the Behavior Checklist.

Behavior Checklist

Name of person under observation _____

Age _____ Observed by _____ staff/family

Recording Scale

0 = behavior not observed
1 = behavior seen 1 or 2 times
2 = behavior seen 3 or 4 times
3 = behavior seen 5 or more times

Behavior	Date	Date	Date
Angry or Agitated	_____	_____	_____
Anxious or Fearful	_____	_____	_____
Clinging to caregiver or others	_____	_____	_____
Cursing and Verbally Abusive	_____	_____	_____
Combative, Hitting, Pushing	_____	_____	_____
Depressed or Sad Mood	_____	_____	_____
Disturbance in Sleeping	_____	_____	_____
Hallucinations	_____	_____	_____
Hoarding Food or Objects	_____	_____	_____
Incontinence	_____	_____	_____
Paranoia	_____	_____	_____
Repetitive Actions	_____	_____	_____
Screaming	_____	_____	_____
Sexually Inappropriate	_____	_____	_____
Territorial Protectiveness	_____	_____	_____

Name two of the most problematic behaviors observed:

1. _____

2. _____

For each problem behavior, answer these questions:

Problem Behavior #1

What time of day does this most often happen? _____

Who else is around or with the resident? _____

What other distractions are nearby? (i.e., television, noise, pets)
_____

Best way to redirect the behavior is_____

Problem Behavior #2

What time of day does this most often happen? _____

Who else is around or with the resident? _____

What other distractions are nearby?
(i.e., television, noise, pets) _____

Best way to redirect the behavior is _____

Other comments or observations: _____

_____

_____

_____

Assessment Summary

Respondent Name _____

Date of Birth _____   Age_____

Location of Assessment _____

Purpose of Assessment:

    ☐ Intake   ☐ Update   ☐ Care Plan   ☐ Reevaluation

Short Portable Mental Status Questionnaire   Score _____
Comments:

Mini-Mental State Exam   Score _____
Comments:

Geriatric Depression Scale   Score _____
Comments:

Other Assessment _____ Score _____
Comments:

Assessment Summary p. 2

During assessment, respondent was observed as:

☐ Cooperative ☐ Hesitant ☐ Agitated

Significant behaviors observed: _____

_____

_____

Recommendations for caregivers or care plan team:

_____

_____

Respondent ☐ is ☐ is not appropriate for group activities

Respondent needs further evaulation by:

☐ Physician ☐ Psychologist ☐ Neuropsychologist

☐ Speech therapist ☐ Physical therapist

☐ Review for case management

☐ Other _____

Signature of Assessor _____

Print Name _____

Assessment Date _____

5

Communication

Communication losses in the stages of memory impairment

The value of nonverbal communication

Twenty ways to communicate more effectively with the memory impaired

Ten communication mistakes

When Messages Are Mixed

"Mother, I can't believe that you bought all these alarms and door guards. There's enough here to secure a bank." Mary looked at the pile of boxes on the kitchen table as if she had never seen them before. "But Bart, you told me that the front door wasn't safe," Mary protested. "I went to a store and the clerk said this was what I needed." "Not just one store, Mother, there are boxes from four different hardware stores." "And besides, I never said you needed an alarm," Bart railed. "What I told you was to call the condominium office and ask for maintenance to repair the screen door. It's not safe to leave the front door open unless the screen door locks securely." Feeling very foolish, Mary sighed, "I guess I forgot again."

Unlike her son, Bart, Mary refuses to "make a mountain out of a molehill." In fact, she recalls that sometimes mix-ups can be fun. Last week, when her granddaughter, Jenna, stayed with her while Bart and

Amy traveled to a convention, Mary prepared Jenna's favorite dinner, spaghetti and salad. As Mary began to serve the meal, Jenna asked, "Gran, where is the pasta?" Mary had carefully marked off every item on her grocery list, but forgot to buy pasta. They both laughed as they checked the refrigerator for alternatives. Finally, they settled down to a new culinary creation, spaghetti sauce over cottage cheese. Jenna pronounced it, "fabulous and really cool." Mary marveled at how Jenna was easygoing like her mother, Amy. Then she warned Jenna, "Don't tell your dad about this, he wouldn't find it funny."

Mary is experiencing communication problems complicated by the onset of "very mild cognitive decline" (Stage 2). When she forgets, she makes a joke about it, like calling herself "the absent-minded grandmother." Recently, Mary confided to a friend that, "the harder I try to remember something, the more I forget." When Mary is stressed, she pushes herself to remember rather than taking a break. That's probably how she ended up with all those alarm devices. Everytime she saw a display with alarms, she connected to the thoughts of "door" and "safe." She misunderstood Bart's original statement and rushed to act. Unfortunately she responded to the wrong message. Between faulty communication and memory lapses, Mary is totally frustrated.

While still in the early stage of cognitive decline, Mary is forgetting directions, confusing word meanings, and experiencing difficulty organizing thoughts. She easily dismisses concern over confusing her son's direction about repairing the screen door. "Bart just didn't make it clear to me what he wanted me to do," she rationalizes away her mistake. "When he gets intense like his father, I just rush to try and do anything to pacify him."

Mary relied on her sense of humor to hide her distress at forgetting to buy pasta for her tried and true spaghetti recipe. She confided to a friend, "I've made spaghetti hundreds of times over the last fifty years and I can't believe I forgot the pasta. Is something really wrong with me? Am I losing my mind?"

Communication Calms Fears

Persons in the earliest stage of memory impairment can feel both depressed and anxious about common mistakes such as those that happened to Mary. One of the greatest fears of senior adults is about becoming memory impaired. Many are widowed, like Mary, and worry about being a burden on their adult children.

If only Mary and others like her would seek help early, they would find a wealth of opportunities. The Alzheimer's Association and specialized memory disorder centers teach practical memory enhancement techniques that work for many older persons.

Mary's desire to live independently and her early stage of memory loss makes her a good candidate to learn memory enhancement techniques. Some health professionals believe that practicing memory enhancement helps some persons delay the progression of memory loss. Whether or not that is accurate, the ability to maintain independence for as long as possible certainly improves the quality of life.

For example, Mary would be taught to reorganize her clothing, kitchen tools, important papers and other frequently used items. Unnecessary or duplicate items are discarded. Clutter is the enemy. Divide into manageable parts and conquer the clutter problem.

Clearly typed reminder cards are placed at strategic locations in the home. Attached to the bathroom mirror might be a card titled, "before going to bed," with reminders to "brush teeth, wash face, take vitamins, turn out the lights." Mary would rely more on recipe cards than on memory when cooking. Her daughter-in-law, Amy, could help prepare a master grocery list with the items most frequently purchased (i.e., milk, bread, juice, cereal, etc.). Mary would note beside these items the number desired, such as: "2 milks, 1 bread." The list is attached to the refrigerator door. Any time Mary thinks of something she needs, she trains herself to write it down immediately.

Mary might also keep a joint calendar with Amy. Each week they can talk about upcoming plans. Amy could help remind Mary of important events such as a doctor's appointment or the bridge club. As Mary checks the calendar or cooks, she speaks aloud to hear herself review each step. These are just a few ways that Mary can again feel in charge of her life.

Gradual Loss of Verbal Communication

Progression through the stages of cognitive decline leads to a regression of receptive language. Communication losses in the early stages of memory impairment are minimal and frequently attributed to fatigue, stress, or anxiety. In the later stages, communication losses are profound as the effects of dementia separate its victims from meaningful contact with the outside world.

The following is a summary of communication losses that are typically experienced at various stages of cognitive decline:

Mild Decline (Stages 2 & 3)

Forgets parts of conversations, directions and requests

Makes irrelevant comments unrelated to discussion

Uses familiar words in the wrong context

Mixes up word order in sentences

Difficulty organizing thoughts

May use repetitive gestures, mixed up words or sounds to fill the verbal void

Moderate Decline (Stages 4 & 5)

Noticeable difficulty recalling names, dates, places, or events

Decreased ability to read and retain information in printed form

Increased frustration in trying to respond to a question, request or direction

Forgets or confuses the meaning of common words

Responds with incomplete sentences or repeated phrases

Severe Decline (Stages 6 & 7)

Gradually loses the ability to recognize spouse, family, friends and caregiver

Verbal communication diminishes and eventually ceases

Extreme difficulty recognizing meaning of words, pictures or any type of symbolic communication

Any remaining language tends to be repetitive phrases or sounds that are not meaningful responses

Unable to understand or respond to directions for bathing, eating, toileting, and other essential activities

Importance of Nonverbal Communication

Imagine traveling to a remote island where the entire native tribe speaks a totally unique language. Their language is not written or diagrammed. They have never heard English, Spanish, French, Japanese, Chinese or any other language except their own. How do you communicate? Nonverbal communication supported by drawing pictures is the only way to transmit ideas between people who cannot speak the same language. For example, draw a picture of a bird. Join thumbs and flutter the other fingers as if to fly. Go outside and point to a bird saying the word, "bird." If the listener makes the connection from these nonverbal examples then the response will be "bird" in that person's language. At least on this one word, the message was sent and received even though the speakers don't have a common language.

Nonverbal communication is equally important in working with the memory impaired. Realize that as the impact of the dementia increases, the memory impaired person can no longer speak or understand the language. Despite these profound verbal losses, a great deal of meaning can be expressed nonverbally. What is commonly called "body language" reinforces or contradicts verbal communication. As the degree of memory impairment increases, body language surpasses verbal language as the primary means of communication.

An observant caregiver learns to read the message in the body language. When a memory impaired resident is clinging or trying to reach out, the need may be for a hug or attention. A resident with clenched fists and eyes darting around frantically, may be fearful or angry. A resident found shaking and trembling appears to be chilled. Another resident pulling at clothing with a strained facial expression probably needs to go to the toilet. An anguished look and an effort to rub or touch the affected area may indicate that a resident is trying to relieve physical pain. Learn to read the message in the actions. This is the body language which is tuned in to basic human needs. Never dismiss unusual body movements as "acting out." Look for the nonverbal message and offer several responses.

Residents in the earlier stages of memory impairment are usually capable of more facial expressions that match feelings of happiness, sadness, fear, pain, or anxiety. As the disease progresses, many sufferers acquire a flat or non-expressive facial appearance.

Family caregivers and facility caregivers can assist others who care for the same resident by making a list (or chart note) of the apparent meaning to certain nonverbal expressions. That information helps others who give respite care or work a different shift to benefit from what is learned about a resident's needs. The more that caregivers communicate on behalf of the resident, the less frustration the resident experiences in trying to get needs met. This is particularly important with respite care or other short term (occasional) caregivers who do not have the time to get to know the resident and his or her habits. Even in a facility with 24-hour staff, the night shift caregivers may not have as much time interacting with the resident as do the day shift caregivers. Simple information such as how a resident calms when humming if the caregiver sings a favorite song can help the night workers be more responsive and consistent in dealing with an agitated, fearful, or distressed resident.

The #1 Principle in Communicating with the Memory Impaired: All caregivers must remember that as long as possible in any way possible a memory impaired person will try to communicate his or her needs.

A final reminder to caregivers, say and show the meaning of any communication with the memory impaired. Approaching the resident who is trembling and appears chilled, a caregiver brings a shawl. First, the caregiver puts the shawl on and shows a smile saying, "warm." Then the caregiver offers the shawl to the resident, helping to place it around the shoulders, repeating "warm" and asks, "are you warm?" A positive expression or cessation of the trembling gives indication that warmth was what the resident sought.

The caregiver's body language and facial expressions are also very important in nonverbal communication. A smile and pleasant voice goes a long way toward calming, reassuring and redirecting a memory impaired person. The opposite is also true. Frustration, anger, and irritation are also clearly expressed by voice and face. The best way to get a positive response is to send a positive message, both verbally and nonverbally.

20 Ways for Caregivers to Communicate More Effectively with the Memory Impaired

The following methods are basic communication techniques that can be used by family caregivers and facility caregivers. No health care experience or college degrees are necessary. These ideas are applicable to novice and veteran caregivers. All that's needed is flexibility, patience, and a willingness to learn by doing.

1. Remain calm.
Impatience and agitation are the sparks that turn confusion into combativeness much like gasoline feeds a fire. No matter how loud or intense the memory impaired person gets, keep a lower tone and speak slowly. To bring calm to a tense situation, the caregiver must model calmness.

2. Make eye contact before giving a direction or asking a question.
Memory impaired persons are easily distracted by sounds and sights around them. Approach the person by calling his or her name, making eye contact, smile, and then begin the direction or question by repeating their name. For example, "Eva." (pause, make eye contact and smile) "Eva, here is your orange juice." or "Eva, do you want orange juice?"

3. Reduce distracting sounds before attempting communication.
Turn down (or turn off) television, radio, and background music. Even the sounds of a dog barking, microwave humming, or another person talking on the telephone can be too much distraction. Close the door or guide the resident toward a quieter room. When too many sounds compete for a memory impaired person's limited attention span, the result can be no response, an uninterpretable response or an aggressive response.

4. Speak directly to the receiver.
Avoid turning away in mid-sentence or calling out from another room. Turning away from the resident gives the message that this person is not important enough to merit the caregiver's full attention. Such a depersonalized approach compounds the resident's confusion about his or her own identity and value. The memory impaired person needs to hear and see the speaker so that nonverbal

and verbal communication combine to carry the message. When the speaker is behind the resident, calling out from another room, or even turned sideways out of view, the memory impaired person has difficulty focusing on the message.

5. Use simple, direct language.
The shortest route to communicating with the memory impaired is to keep it simple and specific. "Tom, sit in this chair." Motion toward the chair and this simple message is complete. "Tom, follow me to the dining room and sit down for lunch." That's a complex message in which the memory impaired person easily gets confused.

6. Give one direction at a time.
Memory impaired persons have difficulty with multi-stage commands. "Sue, put on your sweater, bring your magazine, and wait for me at the front door so we can go shopping." That kind of multi-stage command is total mental overload for the memory impaired. An impatient caregiver may feel ignored or defied. Neither is true. To get a positive response, state each direction separately and allow time for a response. Hand the sweater to Sue and say, "Sue, put on this sweater." (pause) Show the magazine and say, "Sue, do you want your magazine?" (pause) "Follow me to the door." Before opening the door, explain, "Sue ,we are going in the car." Once on the way, say "We are going to the grocery."

7. Repeat a statement or question the same way to avoid confusion.
The resident may not have heard the first time or may need to hear it again to interpret the meaning. "Bill, give the book to me." Repeat this direct statement. If needed, point to the book and hold out a hand to receive it. That's much more effective than following the first request with, "Bill, toss the book on my chair."

8. Check the response to be certain that the meaning is clear.
If the memory impaired person responds with a partial sentence or words that do not match verbal expressions, repeat and check the meaning. Make eye contact and ask, "Are you cold?" "Do you want to go to your room?" Be sensitive to nonverbal expressions and try to isolate exactly what the resident wants.

9. Assist communication by repeating previous statements.

A memory impaired person may speak in partial sentences or be unable to directly express what is wanted. The caregiver repeats what was given and attempts to learn the meaning of what was not stated. For example, if Lettie cries out, "Let me go." First, the caregiver makes certain that she is not being held by another person or otherwise restrained. Then the caregiver observes nonverbal communication and tries to help her complete the meaning. "Lettie, where do you want to go?" "Lettie, do you want to go to your room?" "Lettie, do you want to go to the toilet?" "Lettie, do you want to go outside?"

10. Be a good listener.

A caregiver may be able to listen while doing other tasks. However, the memory impaired person easily loses focus if distracted by the caregiver's movements and activity. Giving total attention to the person who is speaking is a sign of respect. With the memory impaired, good listening is even more important in order to understand the message.

11. A tender touch and open arms can communicate security and acceptance better than words.

A confused, restless or anxious resident seeks reassurance that compassionate contact with another person provides. Be certain that the resident is willing to receive contact. Offer a hand or open arms and move slowly toward the resident's personal space. If rejected, move away slowly and continue to speak comforting words. Never pat a person on the head or shoulders in a condescending gesture. Avoid coming up from behind and touching the resident without first making eye contact.

12. If a resident is in a wheelchair, the caregiver bends down until at eye level before starting to speak.

Bend at the knees and face the resident. Do what is necessary to be "on the same level." Bending from the waist appears as if to loom over the seated person and can be perceived as a threatening posture.

13. Act out the motions of what is being said.

A memory impaired person forgets the steps involved in common activities such as tooth brushing, using a fork to eat, or drinking water from a cup. When the caregiver demonstrates the action while speaking the words, the resident can mimic the action. Sometimes pretending to drink from a cup as an example to show the resident how to drink is too vague. If that does not work, the caregiver needs to actually get a cup of water and drink. Then help the resident bring the cup to the mouth and let the water touch the lips as a cue to drink. Repeating this action several times may be necessary.

14. Show a picture that represents the question.
Make a series of cards that support the meaning of commonly asked questions. Use the picture cards like flash cards that are used to drill multiplication for school children. When asking "Bill, do you want an apple?" show a picture of an apple. Many of the items for flash cards can be cut out from magazines or catalogs, copied from coloring books or simple line drawings. With pictures as communication aids, the resident hears and sees a representation of the question. Adding the pictorial stimuli improves the comprehension potential for some residents.

15. Limit choices to two items to reduce confusion.
For example, as a resident is getting dressed, offer two suitable choices. "Frank, will you wear the blue shirt or the red shirt?" Pause briefly to show each shirt. Follow this process with each item of clothing that involves a choice.

16. If choices are too confusing, work with one item at a time.
As memory impairment becomes more debilitating, the resident can be overwhelmed in trying to eat potatoes, carrots and chicken on the same plate. The way to avoid frustration, fighting and refusal to eat may be to serve each item separately and remove any other nonessential plates or utensils.

17. Give frequent praise and affirmation.
Just getting dressed (even with assistance) is a major task for some memory impaired persons. Remember to give genuine encouragement as each step is accomplished. "Good effort, George." "I knew you could do this yourself." "George, I like the way you are combing your hair."

18. When a resident hallucinates, neither challenge nor criticize.

A resident says that he is being followed by a pack of wild dogs and insists that the caregiver can see them too. Without arguing or challenging the reality of the hallucination, reassure and then attempt to distract the resident's attention elsewhere. The caregiver responds, "Sam, I don't see the wild dogs that you see. But it's ok, because I know how to handle these dogs. Walk with me and we'll find a safe place. Let's go to the sitting room and listen to some music."

19. Before trying to communicate, be certain a resident has eyeglasses or hearing aid working properly.

A memory impaired person may not remember what the hearing aid is or how to use it. The caregiver needs to know how to turn on the hearing aid and how to adjust it. Eyeglasses are easier to use, but just as necessary for some residents.

20. Look for a way to smile in trying situations.

Jacob may have spilled his food again, but at least he didn't throw it. Miriam put her bra on over her blouse and was ready to go outside. If persuasion to correct the clothing fails, ask her to put a jacket on over the outfit. Remember that rock music singers and haute couture fashion designers make fortunes with a similar "fashion statement."

10 Mistakes Caregivers Make in Communicating with the Memory Impaired

1. Demanding attention and action.

A memory impaired person is confused, not defiant. Making demands, shouting, or barking orders will not improve responsiveness or understanding. A calm, encouraging approach with a "we can do it together" spirit is more effective and respectful.

2. Using baby talk.

These residents are adults who have difficulty processing the meaning of language. Baby talk and unfamiliar sounds add even more confusion as well as being demeaning to the person. The resident is more likely to respond to adult language given in slow, simple, one-step requests. Memory impaired persons are not stupid. They are merely losing the ability to access on demand the language, knowledge and experiences of a lifetime.

3. Patronizing speech.

"There, there, dear, it's all right." "You just don't know what's going on, so don't worry about it." " We know what's best for you so don't fight us." The memory impaired person is not comforted by false concern. At the most basic levels, there is a perception of insincerity that may cause the resident to respond with agitation and noncompliance.

4. Insisting on the impossible.

"Tell me why you pulled those books off the shelf." "I told you three times how to brush your teeth, now finish the job." "If you don't tell me what you want to eat, I can't get it for you." Such statements make demands that are beyond the ability of a memory impaired person to achieve. Using contractions such as "don't" are not meaningful to persons in later stages of memory impairment. Memory impaired persons are not able to translate this as "do not." Negative concepts are too obscure. That's why using positive, simple statements are more effective.

5. Shame and blame are never effective.

"I can't believe you did something so stupid." "After the mess you made, I will never take you out to a restaurant again." "Just wait until your son (or daughter) finds out that you refused to get dressed and come to breakfast." Shaming and blaming the memory impaired person for being unable to comply is cruel and demeaning. Even if the words are not understood, the condemning tone is clear. Caregivers would be far less likely to blame a cancer patient for needing help with chemotherapy or shaming a paraplegic for failing to dress without assistance. Memory impairment is a disease that deserves just as much support and empathy from caregivers.

6. Calling out directions from a distance.

The memory impaired person may look up upon hearing his or her name. After that, voices from a distance just blend into the other noises in the environment. Without making eye contact at a reasonably close proximity, the caregiver cannot expect to have the resident's attention.

7. Being critical of the resident who interchanges languages.

When a bi-lingual person becomes memory impaired, expect to hear a mixture of languages. The person may also revert to his or her first language in trying to respond to the caregiver. Don't be critical and demand the resident to "talk to me in English." Ask relatives or another staff member who speaks the language to teach a few simple, comforting phrases in the resident's primary language. Sometimes just hearing a familiar native language is soothing.

8. Shouting at a wanderer to "stop."
A memory impaired person's fears about being threatened or harmed increase when confronted with a loud or angry response. Better to come up alongside the wanderer and talk softly while trying to redirect back to safety.

9. Taking angry words personally.
A combative or agitated memory impaired person strikes out verbally as well as physically to whomever is nearby. The resident who screams "I hate you," even to a loved one is merely giving voice to fear.

10. Telling them who is boss.
Caregiving is about helping an impaired person manage the activities of living as effectively as possible. It's never about control. To be in control assumes that the person being controlled knows to consistently respond to direction. That kind of "control" simply isn't possible with the memory impaired. Caregiving is the wrong type of work for a bossy or controlling person. Effective caregivers are "wellness facilitators," guiding and motivating residents toward independence, self esteem and the greatest possible quality of life.

The Art of Complex Communication

If ordinary communication is an art, then communication with the memory impaired is abstract art. At best, it is a complex type of communication. The meaning is there waiting to be discovered. The forms and images are not always what they seem. The message may require a great deal of interpretation. But there is a message. A skilled caregiver makes every effort to keep the memory impaired person communicating in some way, verbal or nonverbal. At times when least expected, a memory impaired person experiences a "window of opportunity" when he or she really connects with the caregiver in a way that both understand. It's a magical moment that makes all the communication efforts worthwhile.

Joanne is a firm believer in the importance of communicating one-on-one, in whatever means possible with the memory impaired residents in her care. She tells novice caregivers about the time several years ago when she went on a two week vacation. Cal was still able to walk then, although he had lost most verbal communication. The caregiver assigned to him had great difficulty getting him to leave the room in the morning. She couldn't imagine that Cal really liked to take a walk outside as Joanne's reminder note stated.

By the time Joanne returned, Cal was agitated and fighting the two aides who came in to help him dress. She observed the scene from the doorway. Cal was fully clothed but screaming, "get dressed, get dressed." Suddenly Joanne realized what was missing. She walked in and hugged Cal, talking softly to him. Then she went to the closet and brought out his favorite straw hat. "Cal, here is your hat. Put on your hat." With help, Cal put on the hat. Joanne turned him toward the mirror and pointed to the hat, "Now you are dressed. Let's walk." Cal took Joanne's hand and they walked toward the patio.

Knowing Cal's habits, Joanne realized that in order to "get dressed," Cal needed his favorite hat just as much as his other clothing. He was not being resistant to dressing or walking. He was trying to let someone know that he did not feel dressed yet. Joanne received the message because she was a willing listener. Years later, Joanne fondly recalls this "magic moment" of communication anytime she sees a person wearing a tan and brown straw hat like Cal's.

6

Modifying the Environment for the Memory Impaired

Arrangement of interior spaces

Decor Choices

Identification

Exterior Design

Personal Safety

A Safe and Satisfying Environment

"Don't walk on my yard. Go yellow road," Tyronne instructed as his son, T.J., pushed the wheelchair. As they traveled along the brightly painted yellow path, T.J. reflected on how much happier his father has been since moving to the secured memory disorders unit at We Care Village. He found himself humming as a nurse guided another resident along the path singing a familiar song about a yellow brick road.

Just yesterday, T.J. was telling a neighbor some of the things he appreciates about We Care Village. "Eric, one of the activity therapists asked me recently if Dad liked any sports besides track. I told him that Dad enjoyed watching me play college basketball and was always ready for a one-on-one challenge at our makeshift court on the driveway. Next time I went to visit, the nurses aide said that Dad was playing basketball with some guys in the game room. There was

Eric with two teenage volunteers tossing a soft basketball to Dad and three other residents. They were laughing and having a great time. I really had to choke back a tear at seeing Dad get involved in something again. I am so thankful to the staff at We Care Village who keep trying to reach beyond the confusion of Alzheimer's and connect with my Dad as a person."

T.J.'s wife, Shandra, added, "I could hardly go to visit Dad when he was living at City Nursing Center. The hallways and walls were a pale, sickly green that was indistinguishable except for the high shine on the floors. The residents were only allowed to have two pictures on the wall near the bed and very few personal items. The nurse insisted that I take away the brightly colored lap blanket that my Aunt Minnie knitted for Dad. When I questioned it, the director of nursing said that all the residents used only the beige blankets and linens that could be sterilized in the laundry. The staff wasn't even willing to let me bring our dog, Rusty, to visit. Rusty is almost 14 years old, partially blind and incredibly patient. I tried to tell them how Rusty puts his head in Dad's lap while Dad brushes his coat and talks about the times they went hunting together. I'm glad that the people at We Care Village think differently. Rusty is a popular visitor for Wednesday afternoon "Pet Day" as often as I can bring him."

T.J. and Shandra discovered how important a warm, friendly environment is to the well-being of a memory impaired resident. As family members, they also feel genuinely welcome by the staff when they visit. Even their sons notice that Granddad's room "looks like his kind of place." With the blessing of the facility, Tyronne's family decorated his room. The bedspread is an easy care, washable fabric in his favorite color, red. Aunt Minnie's rainbow knitted blanket is draped over the lounge chair. A collection of family photos are on the wall. The wooden tray that T.J. made in junior high shop class is on the dresser. It use to hold Tyronne's watch and state championship ring. Now it holds a pebble, a bingo chip, or whatever Tyronne finds in his pockets. A favorite photo of his late wife, Sue, stands on his bedside table. Shandra had it mounted on a board and varnished so it's sturdy, but without breakable glass. The night nurse says that sometimes she finds Tyronne has fallen asleep still holding Sue's photo in his arms. That thought makes Shandra feel so grateful that Tyronne can live the remainder of his life in a facility that really tries to create a home atmosphere for the residents.

Environment as the Missing Link in Working with the Memory Impaired

Discussions about "environment" in elder care usually relate to the sensitive approach, behavioral initiatives or social activities to promote a sense of community. That is actually the emotional environment. What is frequently overlooked is the importance of the physical environment for memory impaired persons. Whether residing in a facility or at home, the physical environment can help or hinder functioning.

Studies by industrial psychologists have repeatedly demonstrated how productivity in the workplace is diminished by obstacles found in the physical environment. The obstacles may be noise, temperature, equipment, or range of motion. When a correction or improvement is made, productivity increases. Thus the problem was not the inability of the people working in the environment, but rather the problem was the environment.

A similar situation occurs in the environment of the memory impaired. Consider the observation that Shandra made about the main hall areas at City Nursing Center. Walls and floors were a matching shade which she described as "pale, sickly green." The matching colors resulted in one continuous image which creates a depth perception problem for the memory impaired. Residents who cannot discern where the wall ends and the floor begins are more likely to fall or bump into the wall. Add to the perception problem a strong glare from the shine on a highly waxed floor and the area actually becomes a hazard for the memory impaired. A resident who appears to be wandering in such a bland area may be more confused by the lack of visual stimulation than by the memory impairment.

Basic Environmental Design Principles

An environment that fails to support functioning will suppress functioning and increase mobility risks.
A well designed environment for the memory impaired offers safety, comfort, sensory stimulation, socialization, and also encourage mobility.

Specific design adaptations need to be matched to the functional abilities of the residents. Making these changes in a home can be done gradually to correspond with each stage of cognitive decline. Some design adaptations are inexpensive and easy to implement. Other types of remodeling are more costly.

In the last five years, research on the value of environmental design has resulted in the development of state-of-the-art assisted living facilities and skilled nursing homes. What gerontologists have learned about how memory impaired persons interact and react to their environment can be implemented by architects and contractors in adapting the space, design, and decor.

Environmental design that enriches the living space for memory impaired adults works best when implemented as a total concept. This chapter presents ideas for all aspects of living space that can be used to offer cues, ease of mobility, and visual pleasure.

The five areas of importance in creating a suitable and accessible physical environment for the memory impaired are:

1. Arrangement of Interior Spaces
2. Decor Choices
3. Identification
4. Exterior Design
5. Personal Safety

Considering quality of life and potential for mobility, environmental adaptation is a means of accommodating the needs of memory impaired persons that is far less costly than adding more staff or bringing a person into a skilled nursing home before it is medically necessary.

Arrangement of Interior Spaces

The watchwords for interior space in a home or facility are two easy words; clear and simple. In other words, keep the pathways clear of obstacles and the functional space simple. This type of arrangement is probably more difficult to achieve in a home than a facility designed with wheelchairs and walkers in mind. In either situation make a room-by-room review of furnishings, decorator items and pathways that could be hazardous to a memory impaired person.

Designate specific areas for specific purposes.

For example, a dining area in a facility is best used only for meals. Trying to make the dining room do double duty as an activities center or television area adds to the resident's confusion. Whether at home or in a facility, using the dining room as a dual purpose room is an invitation for increased agitated behaviors if the resident expects to eat each time he or she is in that room. Call the room anything you like, even change the sign on the door. Within that room are still the familiar smells, sounds and the routine of sitting down at the tables that relates to mealtime. Expecting the memory impaired person to make the transition is an exercise in frustration for resident and caregiver.

In the home, the caregiver needs to decide whether to serve meals in the dining area or kitchen. Once that decision is made, remain consistent. In years past, a spouse may have enjoyed eating lunch on a tray in the den while watching the noon news, then, in the evening, eating dinner at the kitchen table. Changing locations and adding the distraction of watching television is too difficult for a memory impaired person to manage. The caregiver's best choice for mealtime is a solid table and firm back chair in an area where spills are easily cleaned. Once the choice is made, stay with a consistent location for food service. Don't bring the resident to the table for any other purpose except meals or snacks.

Secure areas with medications, equipment or other potential dangers.

Nursing homes and assisted living facilities generally have adequate security for medication storage rooms. Sometimes less attention is given to medical and cleaning equipment left unattended (even briefly) in hallways or outside the nursing station. Such items as a vacuum, cleaning fluids, or blood pressure stands can become dangers to inquisitive memory impaired persons. In facilities and homes, keep the vacuum and its electrical cord out of walk paths where there's a danger of tripping. If the caregiver must leave the vacuum while attending another person, unplug and stand it close to the wall.

Another danger is available liquids. Cleaning fluids can be spilled, medications mixed up, and both can be ingested causing dire consequences.

The dials and knobs on medical equipment can be very enticing to a resident who just wants to check them out. What often happens in such a case is that medical equipment is damaged or a resident is injured. Take an extra minute to move the items to a secure location or cover with a clean towel to temporarily disguise.

Securing the home for a memory impaired person may leave the other family members feeling that they have to give up their hobbies and interests.

Try storing hobbies and personal items out of reach or in a locked area. For example, woodworking tools must be kept in locked cabinets in a shed or garage. Sewing, crafts, collectibles, computers, or electronic equipment may be transferred to one bedroom that is kept locked. Eliminate the inconvenience of a key lock by installing a screen door hook near the top outside area of the door. Latch the door from the outside when leaving. Unless the memory impaired person witnesses someone opening the latch and copies the behavior immediately, it is unlikely that the resident will be able to open the latch anytime.

Securing potentially dangerous or breakable items benefits everyone in the family. The nonimpaired persons have a secured retreat in which to continue pleasurable hobbies or computer work. The memory impaired person is safe from potential harm.

Disguise or shorten long corridors.

This is a greater problem in facilities than in most homes. A series of doors that all look the same on both sides becomes very confusing for memory impaired persons. In that setting, the emergency exit at the end of the hallway is a powerful lure.

If there is no way to make architectural changes, make cosmetic changes. Paint a garden or backyard scene over and around the door. This effectively disguises the purpose of the door as an exit and makes it part of a total scene. One element, the door, is no longer the most important item in visual range. Place some artificial trees and plants nearby along with a bench. With these inexpensive changes, a dead end hallway becomes a pleasant, sitting area.

Create barrier-free walkways.

Whether in a facility or home, keep pathways to allow the memory impaired person as much independence as possible in walking around living areas. Remove clutter, unnecessary decorator objects, and any breakable items. If wheelchairs are used in the walkways, allow enough room for turning the chair around as well as moving in a straight line.

Remove any decorative glass, full length mirrors, and breakable room dividers.

Place bold decals at eye level and wheelchair level on sliding glass doors. Memory impaired persons have poor depth perception. Don't expect them to remember the difference between the glass door and the solid door. Decorative glass or dividers add to a memory impaired person's confusion when a scene appears to be three dimensional but is actually solid.

If the resident does not understand the purpose of the decals (indicating a glass surface), then add a drape or floor-length blinds to cover the glass door. Only open the drape or blinds when the door is open.

Consider theme areas for easy identification.

A row of ordinary room doors becomes an outdoor scene for a theme unit. A very simple way to implement this is to paint the residents' room doors to look like different types of house doors. Another option is to use the wall space between the doors. On this space, paint windows, landscape, and children playing. With a little paint and a lot of creativity, a bare wall acquires an instant neighborhood feeling.

Give each hallway or unit a different theme. City motifs such as brownstone row houses, the corner grocery and cable cars are familiar to residents who lived in larger metropolitan areas. Another hallway can have a country lane theme with farmhouses, barns, fields of crops, and a cool brook. If possible in a facility, locate residents along the theme hallway which best represents their prior lifestyle (city or country). Other identifying themes can be countries of the world, flowers and trees, or street names. Be creative yet practical. Use themes that are meaningful and easy to identify to the residents.

Decor Choices

When preparing living space for memory impaired persons, put away the fancy magazines and forget the latest fads in furnishings. The best living spaces for the memory impaired are practical, safe, comfortable, and pleasantly stimulating. The following are some tips for achieving this environmental effect.

Avoid floral or small patterned wallpaper.
A memory impaired person cannot tell the difference between violets growing in the yard and the violet pattern on the wallpaper. The resident may damage the wallpaper while trying to "pick the flowers." Small patterns can be perceived as dirt or bugs. For some residents, the preoccupation with the patterns becomes compulsive behavior, frustration, agitation, and finally anger.

Avoid floral, small patterns, or flecks of color in carpets, rugs, drapes, upholstery, and bedspreads.
The same confusion problems arise with these items as with wallpaper. A surprising number of falls and injuries occur when a memory impaired person bends down to "pick dirt off the rug" (small patterns) or pulls down drapes trying to "shake off the lint" (flecks of color). Make certain that a decorator who is selecting these items for a new or remodeled facility takes this very real problem into consideration in selecting fabrics, carpet, and furnishings.

Differing textures are decorative and stimulating to the senses.
Durable, washable fabrics and wallpaper with raised or ribbed textures add to the surroundings for the memory impaired. Be certain that these interesting surfaces are "touchable." Avoid using any textured fabrics or wall hangings in a memory impaired living area that are not suitable for handling and easy maintenance. Washable soft sculptures can be interesting and suitable to touch. Flannel boards with a variety of moveable figures become an interactive picture that can be changed and handled by residents.

Use bold, primary colors on bedspreads, chairs, and to define areas (such as placemats).
Eyesight frequently becomes less acute with aging. A memory impaired person manages better with strong visual cues such as bold colors. A full, rich color attracts attention which can help the resident focus on a task.

For example, the pastel placemats and floral pattern china that has been used in the home for years is no longer appropriate for the memory impaired person. Get a clear tone solid placement in a color that the resident likes. Only use that placement for serving food. Purchase inexpensive, nonbreakable white or beige dishes. The food is easier to find in contrast to the plain plate. The bold color placement provides a frame that draws the eye toward the plate. This is a practical visual cue for mealtime.

Eliminate small throw rugs, large floral vases, and short foot stools.
The potential for injury to a memory impaired person who can trip on these items is not worth the risk.

Select sturdy furniture for common areas.
Sofas and chairs need to be comfortable yet with supportive backs and arms. To create a homelike atmosphere, choose furnishings with colorful, textured fabrics that look like they belong in a living room.

Eliminate delicate chairs or recliners.
The wire "ice cream parlor" chairs or lightweight wicker are not sturdy enough. The open spaces in those designs create difficulty for a memory impaired person trying to distinguish the seat and back areas. Recliner chairs are more difficult to get in and out of than a fixed chair. Also, the mechanism in a recliner contains parts that can pinch or break inquisitive hands.

Put the swivel bar stools (with or without backs) in storage.
This type of seating is not stable enough. A memory impaired person forgets that the seat moves and can easily fall off the stool.

Choose lighting with reduced glare.
Bright lights reflecting off shiny floors and other shiny surfaces cause glare. To the memory impaired person this glare is enough to cause

falls and disorientation to the environment. Diffused or indirect lighting is easier for memory impaired persons to function in than bright lights. Where possible, change light fixtures or use the soft white bulbs.

Use fluorescent lighting only where necessary.
The brightness of fluorescent lights can be toned down with a filtering cover. An important factor with fluorescent light fixtures is to monitor for the humming sound that occurs when not working properly. This sound is irritating to most people and very confusing to the memory impaired. For this reason, some residents have hallucinations more often in areas with fluorescent lighting.

Provide "full spectrum" light bulbs for lamps in community room and craft areas.
These special bulbs were designed in Finland where only a few hours of daylight occur for many months of the year. A full spectrum light simulates daylight, reduces eye strain and promotes a sense of well being. This type of light bulb is more expensive than an ordinary bulb. However, the positive impact can be well worth the cost.

Floor coverings are often overlooked, yet very important in living spaces for the memory impaired.
Carpet is more home-like and reduces noise problems by dampening sound transmission. On the negative side, carpet is never as clean as other types of flooring. Ceramic tile is easier to keep clean and, depending on the style, may not produce glare. Vinyl and some types of tile are also easy to clean but prone to glare and sound problems.

Floor covering is also an important issue for residents who require a walker or wheelchair. Facilities are more inclined to take this into consideration in choosing flooring. The plush carpet that looks so great in the home becomes a hazard as a memory impaired person has a difficulty walking or needs a wheelchair.

The vinyl or tile floors are cleaner and easier for walking devices, but lack the sound-dampening effect of carpet. Large open areas of plain flooring act like a tunnel through which sound can magnify or echo. Greater noise levels are extremely distracting and potentially disorienting to memory impaired persons.

Floor covering must be a solid color that is distinguishable from the wall color.

Keeping to this simple rule is essential to avoid producing depth perception problems for the memory impaired. Borders, stripes or diagonals in the flooring play tricks with perception and result in disorientation.

Identification

Imagine stepping out of the elevator and walking down the hall to look for your room in a hotel. What if every door looked alike with no room number and no other distinguishing features? That's a small glimpse of the everyday confusion that memory impaired persons experience. In many assisted care facilities, bedroom doors usually open onto a central hallway. A series of doors that are the same color and same style are as puzzling to residents as being trapped inside a maze.

Finding ways to help the resident identify personal space is very important. Even in a home, a memory impaired person can wander outside not trying to leave the home but opening the front door instead of the bedroom door by mistake. A family caregiver may be accused by a memory impaired person of "throwing away all my things" if the resident goes into the wrong room.

A personal cue at each resident's door aids room identification.

The cue may be a photo of the resident and the name written in bold, block print. Favorite colors and familiar shapes may also be used in preparing the door identification.

Wayfinding Symbols enhance independent movement.

This is a creative system that uses color, shapes, and symbols as location markers. For example, a sign with a dinner plate, fork and spoon mark the entry to the dining room. Further down the hall, the dining symbol is used with an arrow pointing toward the dining room entry. Long after word recognition is gone, a memory impaired person can associate the plate and utensils with eating.

Daily information boards.

In each main corridor and at the community room, a daily information board displays in prominent block letters the day, date, year, location and season of the year. As a resident stops to look or passes the board, an alert staff member takes note of the resident's interest and starts a discussion about the information on the board. A similar daily board can be created in the home. Set up a marker board with magnets (safer to hold pictures than pins or tacks). Place the daily board in the living room or kitchen where the resident can easily see it.

Special purpose boards.

Similar to the daily information board, the special purpose board highlights weather, holiday information, the daily menu, birthday greetings, or welcome to a new resident. Photos and pictures depicting the theme are excellent. Avoid childish looking cut-outs that belong in a preschool room.

A special purpose board is also excellent for photos of resident activities. Groups, crafts, cookouts, and other events are recognized with photos and names. Many residents enjoy seeing themselves and their names in a place of honor. This is another personal touch that may be used to recognize each resident as a unique human being.

Mark personal belongings.

Using sew-in labels or indelible marking pen, clearly mark all clothing, shoes, and personal items. Particularly in an assisted care facility, labeling is important to insure that personal items are returned to the owner. Sweaters, shawls and shirts are not community property. Show respect for the individual by keeping his or her personal possessions separated from those of other residents.

Exterior Design

Enjoying the fresh air, sounds of birds singing and the warmth of the sun is both pleasurable and healthy for the memory impaired. Access to outdoors is particularly important for persons who have spent much of their lifetimes gardening, farming, or working outside. As delightful as a backyard can be, it also contains botanical and building hazards that must be managed for the safety of the memory impaired.

Verify that all plants and shrubs are not poisonous if eaten.

A memory impaired person may see red berries, confuse them with apples or cherries, and eat them. Make it clear to a landscaper that the area must contain only safe plants without thorns, poisonous elements, or pollen. An excellent source of free advice is the county extension agent.

Soft lighting is needed to define walk paths.
Light also helps to redirect attention to the walking area. In the outdoor areas the problem of bright lights is as much an issue as indoors. Glare or reflections can cause a memory impaired person to become disoriented, thus losing balance and falling or wandering off the walk path.

Locate several sturdy seats along the walk paths.
Wrought iron or wooden benches (with smooth surfaces free from splinters) are good choices for outdoor seating and conversation areas. Place these conversation areas along the walk path for easy access.

In the backyard of a home, put away folding lawn furniture.
This type of lawn furniture is not stable enough and can pinch hands that are tinkering with it.

Provide shade for some seating areas.
Not only is this more comfortable in summer months, but also avoids the confusion of shadows. Persons in wheelchairs or with limited mobility could get a severe sunburn or heat stroke if left unattended too long in the sun. Other residents take certain medications for which too much sun exposure is harmful. With aging, skin becomes more fragile and less resistant to extremes of heat.

Place birdhouses and bird feeders out of reach.
The visual pleasure of watching the birds is very satisfying to some people. Locate the birdhouses and feeders within sight but out of reach. A memory impaired person may try to eat the seeds or dump them out.

Don't hang wind chimes in the garden or outside windows.
To a memory impaired person, the sound of the chimes is confusing and may trigger hallucinations.

Personal Safety

A memory impaired person is constantly trying to explore and relate to the world at large. Curiosity and confusion can lead to accidents and injury. Former awareness of household safety rapidly diminishes. The caregiver in the facility or home must take extra measures to protect the memory impaired person from things so commonplace that a nonimpaired person has difficulty anticipating the dangers.

Cover unused electrical outlets.
Plastic outlet covers are available in hardware stores and the children's section of discount stores.

Remove the dials from the stove.
On most stoves, simply lift the turn dials and place them inside a nearby drawer. By taking this precaution, the caregiver renders it nearly impossible for the memory impaired person to accidentally turn on the stove and create a fire hazard.

Block access to heat surfaces.
Place a barrier around vents, grates, or radiators that can burn. A home alternative is to put a large chair or table in front of the heat surface.

Install a bell or chime to exterior home doors.
An alarm is too frightening. A bell or chime that is loud enough to be heard around the home alerts family that the memory impaired person may be exiting. Several choices for door alarms are available inexpensively in the section of child-proof devices at the hardware or discount stores.

A memory impaired unit in a facility needs an alarm system.
Select an alarm that sounds immediately when the exit door is opened from inside the unit. A quality alarm system will have a matching light panel at the nurses' station to identify which door is opening. To allow unrestricted access by staff, the door alarm can be bypassed by entering a security code on the numerical panel located both inside and outside each exit door.

Remove inside locks from bedroom and bathroom doors.
A memory impaired person can accidentally become locked inside a room. An even better idea is to replace conventional door knobs with easier to open door handles.

Don't use plastic or artificial fruit for wall decorations, centerpieces, or refrigerator magnets.
A memory impaired person cannot tell the difference between artificial fruit and real fruit. Choking and chipped teeth can result. Watch out for holiday decorations that have imitation candy canes or treats as part of the garland. The same concern exists for edible candy, particularly hard candy that is found in candy dishes at home. Hard candy as well as artificial (plastic) candy is a choking hazard.

Limit access to kitchen utensils.
In a facility, the pass-through door between kitchen and dining areas can be locked from the kitchen side during hours between meal service. In a home, install inexpensive child-proof latches on drawers and cabinets. Store cleaners and other chemicals high out of reach or in latched cabinets. Many hazards lurk among common kitchen items.

Install guard rails around toilets and hand rails in tubs or showers.
Memory impaired persons can become unstable on their feet when disoriented. These devices also help the caregiver in keeping the resident supported while attending to basic needs. Medical supply companies provide these devices to fit fixtures in home and facility bathrooms.

Closing Comments on Environmental Awareness

The extent to which environmental conditions influence the behaviors of the memory impaired remains unknown. However, any experienced caregiver knows that clutter, inadequate walkways, poor interior design, and shiny floors create serious problems for the memory impaired.

In evaluating whether a safe and satisfying environment exists in a home or facility, invite several experienced caregivers to tour and make comments. Staff members can engage in an experiential learning opportunity. With a staff partner as an assistant, take turns getting around in a wheelchair and with a walker. Next, take a pair of clear eyeglasses (or buy clear goggles at a hardware store) and smear the lenses with a light coating of transparent cream. Try to walk around looking for environmental cues. The staff partner needs to remain close by to prevent falls. Make an effort to see the world from the viewpoint of a confused older adult with mobility problems. After the exercise is finished, get together with the one or two other evaluation teams to compare notes.

Don't forget to talk with family members. Their insights can be valuable. Perhaps they have ideas that proved effective when the memory impaired person lived at home. Or for the home caregiver, ask persons from the local caregivers support group to help evaluate the home for environmental improvements. Often, a person who is not familiar with the home is more likely to see potential hazards than the people who live there.

Comfortable, safe environments for the memory impaired are the product of sensitivity, awareness, and creativity.

7

Managing Difficult Behaviors

Specific approaches to manage the fifteen common problem behaviors

Triggers for problem behaviors

Caregiver reflections on dealing humanely with problem behaviors

Anger Makes Sense When Nothing Makes Sense

The staff on "B" unit agrees that they can set their watches by Esteban. He arrives every morning at 10 a.m. and stays through lunch. Then he returns promptly at 4 p.m. to help Elena with dinner. This morning, Esteban brings a bouquet of wildflowers. He secretly hopes that she will remember picking wildflowers by the side of the road. That's what they did as they walked home from their first date 54 years ago. Many times they have recalled this special memory. Or maybe the bouquet will remind Elena of how she lovingly braided flowers into headpieces for the wedding of their oldest daughter, Maria. In the years before Alzheimer's disease began to affect her memory, Elena had a special love for fresh flowers.

Esteban whispers a prayer that the emotional outburst yesterday won't happen again. He hopes that they can just sit together on the patio holding hands. For a while after lunch, Elena is calm and listens to Esteban read letters from their grandchildren. Suddenly, without warning, she throws the flowers and screams, "Go away, you are trying to kill my Esteban, go away!" Esteban and a staff member follow her down the hallway trying to reassure her that he is here and he is safe. He holds out his hand. She pushes him aside saying, "I hate you. I only love my sister Carmen." Once again, tears well up in Esteban's eyes as he watches his wife of 52 years reject him for Carmen, a hallucination.

As he walks out toward the lobby, Alma Drew, the social worker invites him to come to her office for a cup of coffee. She reminds Esteban that Elena does not realize what she is saying in this stage of severe cognitive decline. In his mind he knows what Alma says is true, but her words can't mend his heartache. He confides in Alma, "I could handle her confusion, her forgetfulness and her fears. I don't know how much longer I can listen to her harsh words. My Elena was never a bitter or spiteful person before this disease. I just can't reach her anymore."

Like many family members, Esteban thought he could cope with anything the disease brought into his life. The Alzheimer's Family Support Group gave him many useful ideas for dealing with Elena's difficult behaviors. He tried most of them and some actually worked for awhile. But not anymore. Esteban notices that even the staff in the memory impairment unit is having less success in redirecting Elena's attention when she screams at him.

Esteban is finally ready to admit that even a deep love for his wife is not enough to erase the pain of her rejection. He can't understand why she is angry. Elena is safe, not in physical pain and receives much encouragement from the staff in the memory impairment unit. He adjusts his life around spending time with her daily. In despair, he says to Alma, "I suppose that for Elena, anger makes sense when nothing else makes sense."

Managing Problem Behaviors of the Memory Impaired

Whether functioning as a family caregiver or a staff caregiver, the stress of dealing with a memory impaired person's anger, abusive actions, or false accusations becomes very heavy to bear. Direct care providers are in the line of fire, sometimes literally, as objects are hurled at them. Add to that the harsh words and lack of gratitude from the memory impaired persons who need help and a picture emerges of the daily stress-laden challenge of caregiving in the home or a facility.

Many caregivers lack the resources and training to understand how much the disease affects behaviors. "Taking it personally" only makes the job more stressful. Even the most dedicated gerontologists have to make an effort to separate their feelings for the person from their discomfort with the problem behaviors. Family and facility caregivers who are in most direct contact with memory impaired persons need strong commitment and love for this work in order to deal with the stress and confusion that is expected in dealing with problem behaviors. Because this issue is so important, a later chapter is devoted to managing caregiver stress.

An introduction to the typical problem behaviors of memory impairment was presented in Chapter 2. Recall the key definition of a "problem behavior":

A problem behavior interrupts functioning in a way that endangers the safety of the individual or other persons in the environment.

This chapter moves beyond identifying the problems to offering answers that direct care providers can use in working with the memory impaired. In the sections that follow, suggestions are offered for managing the common problem behaviors associated with memory impairment.

Whatever techniques that a family caregiver or facility caregiver decide to use, consistency is crucial to success. The best way to learn positive behavior management techniques is through repetition. Consistency helps the caregiver develop automatic responses that are affirming, encouraging, and set appropriate limits. Consistency also reduces the potential for over-reacting to behaviors that can be irritating or threatening.

Along with consistency, the next most important characteristic for caregivers in dealing with problem behaviors is flexibility. Accept the reality that a memory impaired person's behaviors are unpredictable. At times, redirecting a problem behavior can be as simple as singing a favorite song or giving a reassuring touch. Other times, the caregiver must try several approaches before engaging the resident's attention or confidence enough to interrupt the problem behavior.

In managing problem behaviors, caregivers are like detectives. The behaviors are "clues" that lead to identifying the real "culprit." Good observers discover "suspects" along the way. Anxiety, fidgeting, shaking and restlessness are "clues." Looking around the area, the caregiver sees some "suspects"; an open door (noise or temperature), several residents crowding together on the sofa (need for closeness, protecting territory) and the anxious resident is sitting beneath the air conditioner vent (cold air, noise). The caregiver's "deduction" is that the resident is cold and cannot find the words to express the need for warmth. After closing the outside door, the caregiver brings a sweater for the resident. An accurate deduction results in a reduction of problem behaviors.

Specific Responses to Problem Behaviors

Caregivers learn quickly from daily experience how to recognize the problem behaviors. A typical concern of caregivers is, "what do I do next?" In an effort to answer that question, caregiver responses are presented for fifteen problem behaviors that are common to memory impaired persons.

Make a note of suggested responses that work well. Facility staff follow established procedures for chart notes. Also be sure to pass along this information to the treatment team and staff on the next shift. Family caregivers need to keep an informal chart, or just a notebook, with similar caregiving notes. Share these response methods with other persons who may spend time with the memory impaired relative such as other family members, adult daycare workers or respite care staff.

Anger

Remain calm and alert
When a memory impaired person is angry, he or she may suddenly become loud, belligerent, or aggressive. Even experienced caregivers can feel fearful and threatened by such behaviors.

Manage your responses before you address the other person
Family members who are just beginning to be caregivers can be shocked, stunned, or defensive at such outbursts. Getting beyond

these natural responses is very important. Keep repeating silently, "the disease is causing these behaviors."

Never force or intimidate
Above all, avoid the mistake of trying to meet force with force. The memory impaired person is likely to become more agitated and resistant if the caregiver responds aggressively.

Remove distractions
Look first for the basic sources of distraction which might provoke an angry or confused response. Turn off the television or radio. Close the outside door or window. Send noisy pets outside. Ask other persons to move away from the angry resident or gently guide the resident to another room.

Acknowledge the anger
Say aloud that you recognize the resident's anger and that you are here to help. Take time to make eye contact and give genuine assurance of your interest. Avoid questioning ("what do you have to be angry about?") or diminishing the intensity of resident's feelings ("that's not such a big deal").

Maintain eye contact and use a moderate voice tone
Regardless of your frustration as a caregiver, keep a moderate to low tone of voice and casual pace. Rapid fire speech and shrill voice tone does nothing to soothe an angry person. Maintaining eye contact sends the nonverbal message that you are listening.

Redirect attention
Try to redirect the resident's attention by offering alternatives (i.e., food, drink, singing together or taking a walk). Choose an alternative that is usually well received by the resident. Encourage but do not force a choice.

Remain until the behavior changes
Allow time for the resident to de-escalate from the anger. Redirection followed by a rapid retreat often leads to a more intense anger outburst later. If the caregiver cannot remain, try to get the resident involved in an activity with another resident or family member.

Anxiety

Scan the surroundings

Look for obvious sources of distress (i.e., noise, strangers, new clothing, or furniture moved). Try to determine what is occupying the resident's attention.

Affirm concern

Tell the resident that you realize there is a problem and you are here to help. Demonstrate with your full attention that you are here to help.

Offer comforting contact

If the resident is willing, extend your hand or offer your arm to hold while walking. Some residents resist personal contact. Instead present a soft pillow or stuffed animal to hug.

Guide away from sources of distress

A typical example involves room noises in a crowded restaurant or dining room that prompt anxiety. Take the resident to a different table in a quieter section or leave the dining area. Many anxiety reactions are the result of excessive stimulation.

Speak in a calm, reassuring manner

Get close enough to be heard without invading personal space. Speak slowly and clearly. Restate the concern within a helpful context ("I see that you are afraid. I can help you. Please come with me to the living room.")

Clinging

Pause from activity and talk with the resident

Clinging is a sign of insecurity. The resident needs to know that the caregiver is aware of his or her presence. Spend a few moments talking with (not talking at) the resident.

Find a task to occupy the resident while the caregiver completes other work

Ask the resident to help with a simple task, such as folding, dusting, or arranging clothes in a drawer. Seat the resident in visual range of caregiver working area or just outside the room (i.e., family caregiver wants privacy for a bath). If out of visual range, sing or speak occasionally to remind the resident that you are near.

Engage the resident's attention
In a facility, the caregiver can guide the clinging resident to an activity group or bring in another resident and give them a task to do together.

Offer a comforting substitute
When the caregiver must leave the home or move on to attend another resident, give the clinging resident a special task. For example, ask the resident to take care of a stuffed animal or baby doll until you return.

Cursing

Avoid being judgmental or feeling insulted
Cursing is not limited to persons who cursed before memory impairment. Family members are stunned to hear prim and proper grandmothers shout profanities that would make a drunken sailor blush.

Cursing is a "clue," not a problem
A memory impaired person curses out of frustration and inability to find the right words to express feelings or needs. Caregivers are more effective when they focus on finding and dealing with the source of the distress.

Cursing may be a predictor of combativeness
For some memory impaired persons, cursing leads to combativeness as distress increases. Smart caregivers recognize this pattern and attempt to de-escalate the situation before violent behaviors occur.

Take the resident away from a crowd or possible ridicule in a public place
The attention given to the cursing resident can increase the frustration or reward the behavior. Guide the resident to a quiet room or step outside (or in the hallway) of a public place. Approaches used in responding to anger or anxiety can be used to redirect the resident.

Combativeness

Observe the times and places

Frequently, combativeness is a response to direct care. For example, the only time a resident may kick or hit is during showers, changing clothes or combing hair. The confused resident may feel attacked or cornered. Go slowly and give repeated reassurance.

Slowly back away a few steps.

Break the tension by moving away, like a boxer stepping out of the ring. Give the resident as much freedom of space as is safe. This places the caregiver out of kicking or slapping reach. Be quiet or speak in a low, calm tone. As you try again to approach, place arms at your side in a nondefensive posture.

Don't try to hold the resident unless safety demands action

Never restrain or wrestle with a resident unless he or she is in immediate physical danger. Call for staff assistance. In homecare, call a neighbor or dial 911 to get help from paramedics. When the confused person is throwing things, cover face with a shield (i.e., sofa cushion, laundry basket) or get behind furniture.

Use your voice for comforting instead of touch.

As the confused person begins to calm down, don't rush to hug or touch. This gesture can be mistaken as a restraint and trigger another aggressive episode. Positive words of reassurance are the safest means of comforting.

Depressed Mood

Spend time with the resident

The sad facial expression and isolation from others are indicators of a depressed mood that needs attention from the caregiver.

Determine if the resident is lonely, bored, or in pain

If the depressed mood improves when other needs for companionship are met, then the resident's behavior is merely a "clue" to another problem. A continuing sad mood may be related to physical pain or discomfort.

Ask the resident to talk about favorite subjects
Reminiscence (or recalling memories) is a simple yet powerful way to use positive past experiences as a source for strength to cope in the present. Telling stories from the past are not just meaningless ramblings. Use what is learned from these reminiscences to praise the resident's positive qualities and achievements.

Be alert for medication changes
Changes in medication, dosage, or conflicts with over the counter drugs can result in dramatic mood changes. Depressed mood can be another "clue" to medication related problems. At home, check the medicine cabinet for accurate doses and schedule.

Can a person with dementia be depressed?
Some physicians do not believe that persons with dementia can be depressed. However, a substantial amount of geriatric research contradicts that belief. National Institutes of Health report advocates assessment and treatment of geriatric depression. If the primary physician will not listen to the caregiver's concerns, get a second opinion or bring in a geriatric psychiatrist.

Take seriously any talk of self-harm
Never assume that a memory impaired person can't cause a self inflicted injury. Alert the primary care physician immediately. Seek psychological assessment and counseling as additional responses to this concern.

Disturbed Sleep

Follow a routine leading to bedtime
At least half hour before bedtime, turn off television and reduce activity level. The routine signals bedtime.

Leave on a night light or soft music
A memory impaired person who awakens confused becomes more fearful in a dark room. Choose instrumental music or a music box. The announcers and commercials on a radio station add to the confusion and sleeplessness.

Do light stretches or take a walk

Light exercise can help relax the body for sleep. Residents who nap frequently in the afternoon or have little physical activity are not as likely to sleep through the night. A short easy walk helps some residents prepare for sleep.

Limit types and amounts of liquids

Within two to three hours of bedtime, reduce the intake of beverages with caffeine such as tea, chocolate, cola, and coffee. Offer decaffeinated drinks or find substitutes. Consult with the physician about the limitations that are best suited to each resident.

Get a physician's evaluation

Sleep disturbance can be a side effect of medication (or certain medication combinations), symptom of depression, or related to a physical problem.

Hallucinations

Never challenge the resident's "reality"

Hallucinations are "real" to the resident. What the resident claims to see, hear or feel is an honest response. Arguing that point does nothing to improve the resident's feelings of calm and security.

Check for environmental "clues"

Look for glare, lights or background noises. As explained in the chapter on modifying the environment, these elements can trigger or sustain hallucinations.

Change locations

Guide the resident to another room, into the hallway, or outside. Changing locations breaks the intensity and may remove the resident from the irritating stimuli.

Give frequent and appropriate assurances

With a positive tone, remind the resident, "Whatever upset you, I am here to help" or " I am with you." Offers of comfort and companionship are more effective then platitudes like, "there's nothing here to worry about."

Use a distraction

Offer a light snack or drink. Open a picture book and begin asking which picture the resident likes. Start to sing a favorite song. Try to engage the resident's attention on a topic that is pleasurable and safe.

Schedule medical evaluation

Hallucination can result from infections, pain, dehydration, alcohol abuse, or medication reactions. A medical examination is important to identify or eliminate these treatable conditions as triggers for hallucinations.

Schedule a vision exam

If no medical reasons are found for the hallucinations, the resident may actually be having trouble seeing what is really there. Changes in visual acuity, cataracts, glaucoma, or reduced depth perception may account for what seems to be hallucinations.

Hoarding Food or Objects

Remove valuable items

The memory impaired resident is not stealing, more likely the resident picks up interesting objects to examine, sort, or put away. Shortly thereafter, the resident forgets both picking up and relocating the items. Avoid leaving purses, money, jewelry, or other valuables in sight and reach.

Designate a secure space

Find a high shelf, locked cabinet, or other location for storing personal items of staff or guests. A place that is out of sight or locked discourages hoarding. A simple child-proof latch allows easy, keyless access for caregivers.

Notice frequently used hiding places

Commonly used hiding places are sofa cushions, under the bed, open containers, and trash cans. It's not so much that the resident remembers the hiding place as that it is easily accessible within the resident's routine activities.

Limit food service to one area

Serve all food in the dining area. Avoid giving the resident a snack to take to another room.

Plan ahead for critical items
Home caregivers: have spare keys and eyeglasses.

Avoid shaming the resident
The resident is confused and forgetful, not dishonest or defiant. Blame the disease, not the individual.

Incontinence

Establish toilet routines
Take the resident to the bathroom at regular intervals. As much as possible, find toilet times that fit the resident's habits. Be sure to toilet before bedtime or transporting to another place.

Limit liquid intake 2 -3 hours before bedtime
Reducing the need to awaken and toilet means less accidents and less sleep disturbances.

Respond rapidly to nonverbal clues
Typical clues are pulling at clothing, pacing, painful facial expressions, or anxiety.

Use environmental clues
Place a photo of a toilet on the bathroom door. Some residents are able to respond to the toilet photos with arrows pointing to the way as cues for finding the bathroom.

Clear the bathroom of distractions
Remove unnecessary objects, decorator items and magazines if they distract the resident. At home, be certain that medicine cabinets are locked.

Reduce opportunities for toileting mistakes
A memory impaired person may confuse a decorator vase, antique wash bowl or other open object as a toilet and use it for that purpose.

As with other problems, avoid shaming
The progression of the disease causes the resident to forget when, where, and how to handle toileting needs. Praise toileting successes. Show acceptance of the accidents and respect toward the person.

Handle public accidents calmly

Take the resident to the bathroom or a private room to clean up as much as possible. Don't be timid about asking for a mop or cloths in a public place. Apologize for any inconvenience but don't feel guilty. Remember, this is a consequence of the disease, not a deliberate misbehavior.

Paranoia

Access the situation

The basic techniques previously described for dealing with hallucinations are applicable with this problem. Of primary importance is not to over-react no matter how odd or offensive the resident's claims may be. Don't allow staff or family members to ridicule or take lightly the resident's behaviors and fears.

Make an effort to be helpful

Offer to help the resident look for missing things. Complaints about missing personal items are sometimes valid. The items may be misplaced by a forgetful resident or moved by someone else. Another resident may be hoarding and hiding the items. Do not assume the resident is wrong or rush to label the behavior as paranoia.

Accept the fear without affirming the paranoia

Many memory impaired persons fear "losing things." Looking for items seems to be a metaphor for the real problem, losing memory and mental processes. Recognize the fears as real, regardless of whether the reason for the fear is logical. For example, say to a resident, "I know you are afraid of robbers, but I've never been robbed here. If any robbers come here, I'll protect you." Give ample reassurances that the location is secure and that you are genuinely concerned about the resident's safety.

If accused of theft, don't argue.

Trying to reason with a confused person leads to more agitation and possible combativeness. Call another staff member or neighbor to assist. Let the second person calm the resident while the accused person leaves quietly. In a facility, report the incident to the staff supervisor. Follow procedures to protect resident rights. Unfamiliar persons and places as well as crowds becomes overwhelming to a person with paranoia. Acting out behaviors are more likely to occur with these exposures.

Repetitive Actions

If the behavior is not harmful, ignore it
Repetitive rocking, clapping, tapping, or folding may be soothing to the resident. Since these actions are not harmful, let them continue until the resident moves on to something else. Other repetitive actions such as picking a wound, public masturbation, pulling out hair or head banging do need redirection.

Offer a suitable substitute
Practical substitutes are a small squeeze ball, modeling clay, and folding clothes.

Encourage movement; a walk or light stretching
Movement interrupts the repetitive actions with healthy activity as the distraction.

Make eye contact and start a conversation
The repetitive actions may be clues to boredom and isolation. Personal attention and socialization can interrupt the repetitive cycle. Attempt to involve the resident in a group activity.

Increase sensory stimulation activities
Repetitive actions can be a "clue" that the resident seeks sensory stimulation. Kneading dough, sand trays, fabric texture sorts, and other sensory stimulation exercises work well.

Screaming

Search for the message
A late stage memory impaired person may scream due to inability to verbalize words or sentences. A person who still has usable vocabulary is likely to scream in response to situations or frustration.

Look for potential sources of fear
Changes and inconsistency often result in a fear reaction. What is new or different in the environment?

Note the times and places screaming occurs

Identifying these factors leads to discovering possible sources of distress. Usually the caregiver can work around these factors to reduce the resident's fears and screaming. For example, the resident may fear the noise of the vacuum cleaner and scream at the person who is cleaning. Arrange for the resident to be elsewhere when the vacuum is used.

Respond without over-reacting

Check for problems or distress. Avoid babying or putting down the chronic screamer. Screaming is attention getting however, more attention may be what is needed.

Sexual Inappropriateness

Guide the resident away from public view

Remember that this person has forgotten the social rules about sexuality that prohibit masturbating or fondling self through clothing in public. Without calling more attention to the behavior, take the resident away from a group to avoid ridicule.

Offer a suitable distraction

Give the resident a stuffed toy to hug to keep the hands occupied appropriately while the caregiver attempts to gain the residents attention. Talk about the resident's positive qualities; "I really like to see your smile. I think you are very special."

If touched inappropriately, don't overreact

Gently remove the resident's hands from your body and step slightly away from reach. Begin to talk about something else to redirect the resident.

For caregivers who have been sexually abused in other circumstances, this situation will be extremely difficult. Adult children who are sexually touched by a memory impaired parent usually feel horrified and betrayed. Make an effort not to transmit personal distress to the memory impaired person who is not aware of the implications of the action. Any caregiver who is emotionally distressed by the resident's behaviors needs to seek counseling to avoid allowing this incident to cause further harm.

Territorial Protectiveness

Approach personal items with respect

Remember that the memory impaired person's world is what is in sight and close range. Forgetfulness can prompt the unconscious need to gather, hoard, and hold personal possessions. Always ask permission to move or rearrange the resident's personal items.

Caregivers are referees and diplomats

When a resident fights for a certain seat or claims a property of others, rearrange or remove the coveted object.

Lead away from the coveted area by another route

For example, a resident refuses to allow table mates to sit down. Invite him or her to help you get more napkins. Walk around briefly. Return the resident to the table. The tension is often broken by the distraction.

Encourage joining a group activity

Staking out territory is a type of social isolation. Bring the resident to a neutral territory (location of the group activity) and redirect attention on the activity instead of the place.

Give more reassurances and attention

The resident may be trying to communicate insecurity. Show more personal attention. Offer a hand to hold or a hug, if the resident is willing.

Triggers for Problem Behaviors

Just as the flash of lightening occurs before the crashing sounds of thunder, certain triggers (persons, places, events) are often seen in advance of problem behaviors. Recognizing the most common potential triggers eases the caregivers work and ultimately benefits the memory impaired person with more positive caregiver attention. The triggers are not necessarily the cause of problem behaviors in memory impaired persons. However, if left unchecked, the triggers can exacerbate problem behaviors. The following points may trigger a variety of problem behaviors.

Over-stimulation

Too much noise or activity aggravates confusion, paranoia, and anger in memory impaired persons. Even therapeutic activities can be counterproductive if not balanced with time to relax. Visitors, travel, eating at restaurants, and holidays are prime examples of good things with the potential for over-stimulation for a memory impaired person.

Under-stimulation

The blank expressions and listlessness seen in some memory impaired residents are the results of not enough useful stimulation. Sometimes the problem is insufficient caregiving personnel. Other times the problem is poor attitudes among staff who choose to be caretakers, meeting minimal needs.

Separation Anxiety

Moving from home to an assisted living facility takes away familiar sights, sounds and routines. The environment and the people are foreign to the new resident. Cues used to get around a well known location (home) are now missing. Expect an adjustment period for new residents (and those moving to a different unit or room) to be filled with anger, confusion, anxiety, fear, insecurity, and acting out behaviors that may be different than those previously observed.

Change in routine

Consistency is important in care of the memory impaired. Even positive and necessary changes in routine take time to establish. Until the new approach becomes the routine, many residents will have adjustment problems. Changes that are mere interruptions need to be monitored and corrected.

Physical discomfort

Illness, both major and minor, can heighten the resident's confusion and frustration. The inability to verbalize symptoms, pain or physical problems leaves memory impaired persons with trying to get attention any way possible (i.e., screaming, acting out, anger, aggression). Sudden or extreme behavior changes may also be a clue to the caregiver that there is an undetected physical problem occurring (i.e., fever, constipation, aches, dehydration).

Medication reactions

Anytime changes are made in the memory impaired person's medication, watch for possible behavioral problems. Too much or too little medication can create physical or emotional distress. Check the literature that comes with the prescription for a listing of potential medication reactions. Medication reactions may include apathy, depressed mood, sleep disturbances, excessive sleep, agitation, hyperstimulation, paranoia and hallucinations. A new medication or a combination of medications are prime "suspects" when the "clues" involve sudden increase of problem behaviors. Report any potential reactions or other notable behavior changes to the prescribing physician immediately.

New caregivers

Changes in primary caregivers or favorite caregivers can result in extreme behavioral responses. When a spouse/caregiver takes a vacation or a caregiver quits the job, the memory impaired person is like a ship tossed about without its anchor. Considering that caregivers assist with very personal activities (i.e., bathing, toileting, dressing), the resident may resist the presence of a stranger in this role.

Hostile environment

If the caregiver is angry, loud, demeaning, or neglectful, the resident is more likely to act out as a defensive response. Even hostility that is within the environment, but not directed at the resident can cause distress. Examples of this situation might be family members arguing outside the resident's door or one caregiver shouting directions at a coworker. A confused person who does not clearly understand the reasons for hostility cannot be expected to respond appropriately.

Personality traits

Every member of the caregiving staff needs to read the social history of each memory impaired resident. The same kind of information needs to be given by family caregivers to neighbors or extended family who will be helpers or relief workers in contact with the memory impaired person. Certain personality traits are enduring, even in dementia. For example, a person who has always responded to frustration, discomfort, or change with an explosive temper is more likely to become aggressive than a person with an even-tempered, kind nature.

Occasionally the disorientation and fear that accompanies memory loss may cause a formerly calm person to become angry, suspicious, or isolative. Positive therapeutic techniques and enlightened caregiving can help these people reconnect with the gentleness that has been their lifelong nature. Unfortunately, the aggressive, bitter, critical personalities rarely become gracious and charming after the onset of dementia.

Progression to another dementia stage

The transition between stages of dementia as representative of cognitive and skill losses is not a clear cut "here today, there tomorrow" distinction. Repeated changes in behaviors, dislikes of things formerly liked, and reduction in communication skills are "clues" that the resident is entering another stage in the disease process.

Walking the Mile

In summary, both caregivers and memory impaired persons are affected by problem behaviors. No one wins, unless they all win. Think about the old folktale that advises never to criticize anyone until you've walked a mile in their shoes. Since there is no reliable predictor of who will become a victim of memory impairment in the future, today's caregiver could someday become a resident of the same dementia care unit. Adult children as caregivers of a memory impaired parent demonstrate attitudes that may be used toward them someday. In the most trying and frustrating moments, consider these questions:

How would I want to be treated?

How much respect for personhood, privacy and preferences is suitable?

If I could not manage my own behaviors, is it fair to hold me responsible?

If I felt lost, confused and trapped in a strange existence, would I scream, cry, or flail to try to make connection with another human being?

As a memory impaired person, would I deserve less consideration and caregiver attentiveness than a person with cancer or paralysis?

Looking at these questions from the viewpoint of the memory impaired person can be very enlightening. Follow the wisdom of scriptures and "do unto others as you would have them do unto you." That is the golden rule for all caregivers.

8

Memory Impairment is a Family Issue

The REAL changes that memory impairment brings to a family

When home caregivers yield to professional caregivers

Connecting with a support system

"Welcome to the annual Centerville Conference for Caregivers of the Memory Impaired. My name is Doris Elgin. I'm the chairman of the Midtown Memory Impairment Family Support Group. This conference touches my life because I'm a nurse who has worked in the memory impaired unit at We Care Village until three years ago when my husband, Bruce, was diagnosed with Alzheimer's disease. Now I'm a full-time home caregiver. Whether you are a family caregiver or part of a caregiving staff, this conference has something for everyone. In addition to hearing our panel of speakers, take time to network with other families and caregivers."

There is no doubt as to why Doris is one of the area's most popular speakers on caring for the memory impaired. Her sparkling personality and positive outlook demonstrate that families can survive memory impairment. Beyond that, Doris is an enthusiastic advocate of enlightened attitudes of caregiving.

Sitting in the audience, Amy is taking notes while her husband, Bart, repeatedly excuses himself to make business calls. After an hour, he announces that "this isn't useful to us," picks up his briefcase and leaves. At the coffee break, the attractively dressed woman sitting next to Amy says, " I didn't think it applied to my mother either, but finally I came to realize that it does. By the way, my name is Adrienne."

"My name is Amy, and it's my mother-in-law that I'm worried about. But my husband, Bart, just refuses to think of his mother as having any problems except disorganization."

Finding a common bond of concern, Amy and Adrienne continue their conversation during the conference lunch break. Adrienne shares all the symptoms that she tried to ignore before a crisis led to taking her mother, Vivien, for assessment. Amy is so relieved to hear another family member's view about what to expect in an assessment appointment. She admitted being afraid that Mary would be subjected to painful medical tests or locked up in a psychiatric ward. Talking to other families is giving Amy a completely different view of dealing with a memory impaired loved one.

At the close of the conference, Amy purchased an audio tape of the presentation given by T.J. and Shandra. This young couple spoke about a subject that addressed Amy's fears: how to choose the right caregiving facility for a family member and how to know the time to make the move. Amy wants Bart to listen to how T.J. spoke of his difficulty in accepting the diagnosis and how he tried to push his father to do things beyond his abilities. T.J. talked about learning to see a different kind of strength in his father, one that did not depend on performance or success. Shandra spoke openly about the arguments they had before T.J. accepted his father's limitations. She also told of situations in which her entire family, including their teenage sons, became closer by working together to maintain communication with their grandfather. Before leaving, Amy thanked Shandra and T.J. for their inspiring words and shared briefly why it was so meaningful. T.J. offered his business card to give to Bart, "ask him to call me for breakfast sometime and we'll talk son to son about facing our parents' needs." On the way to the car, Amy waved at Adrienne, Doris, and several other ladies she met during the conference. No matter what Bart does, Amy plans to attend the Midtown Memory Impairment Family Support Group. If she learned anything today it's that memory impairment is not just her mother-in-law, Mary's problem. It's a family issue that requires a family response.

Shaking the Family Tree

Memory impairment changes a family forever. It shakes, bends and sometimes causes breaks in the family tree. From the onset of symptoms through assessment and care planning, every family touched by memory impairment experiences significant changes. These changes are REAL and involve these real areas of life:

Relationships
Economics
Activities
Location

Let's look at how these REAL changes affect the lives of a family with a memory impaired loved one.

Relationship Changes

The relationship changes that impact the balance of power are more notable as the degree of functioning declines.

The self-reliant husband who formerly took pride in protecting his wife, must now be dependent on and protected by her. He loses personal power as she loses the security of being cared for in order to care for him. They are both depressed and confused. He has Alzheimer's disease. She grieves for the loss of her spousal role and what she believes is the end of their idyllic retirement lifestyle.

The formerly active grandmother whose high energy and talent for arranging special events made her home the center for family fun, is now being shuffled between three adult daughters for caregiving. At different stages of parenting (empty nest, teens and toddlers) the daughters are equally resentful at the four-month intrusion into their schedules that occurs during their "turn to manage mother."

A retired military officer forgets everything but his ability to bark orders. He argues with his son, criticizes the grandchildren, treats his daughter-in-law like a maid, and constantly tries to kiss the neighbor whom he thinks is his wife. Accustomed to "taking orders from the Commander," this family yields to old patterns that dementia has rendered unhealthy for everyone.

Family relationships are never the same after memory impairment. The changes are felt throughout the family for two (victim/children) or three generations (victim/children/grandchildren).

Love and dislike can exist simultaneously

Some family members retreat emotionally, then literally, as the loved one sinks further into dementia. Families become divided between those who accept and those who don't accept the disease.

Gaylene's sister and daughter actually tell people that she is dead. To them, her personality is gone and nothing is left but a "droopedshoulder woman who insists on dressing like a bag lady and wearing those ridiculous socks." Gaylene spent most of her life as a fashion model; tall, proud, stylish, and beautiful. She trained and helped launch her niece, Sarah, into a successful modeling career. Between world travels and photo sessions, Sarah visits the nursing home as often as possible. When she visits, she brings an overstuffed tote bag of supplies for their "beauty day." Sarah gives Gaylene a facial, paints her nails and brings a bright new silk hair bow. To Sarah, Gaylene is still beautiful. Everytime Sarah visits, the nurses are certain that Gaylene stands taller, smiles more and moves with a gracefulness that comes from being surrounded by love.

Jane never knows "what man will wake up next to her." One day Jacob is quiet and follows her around like a shadow. He just "wants to be close." On those days, they can cuddle and enjoy being together. He hardly talks, yet he looks at her with love like the old days. Another day it's "Jacob the terrible." He screams and curses at Jane. He insists that she is allowing strangers to come into their home and steal his "hidden treasure." Jane has no idea what "hidden treasure" means and she certainly wouldn't invite anyone into the house when he is in a rageful mood. She sings, she prays, she tries to scrub away her frustrations. By late afternoon, she daydreams about all she could be doing if Jacob were dead. Later that night when he finally falls asleep, Jane feels guilty about wishing for his death.

Every family member must choose his or her reaction to the memory impaired person. Gaylene's closest relatives deny the truth and avoid contact. Either they are ashamed of what the disease has done to her former physical attractiveness or they are not willing to help even minimally in her care. Sarah's genuine love and respect for her aunt is greater than any ravages of the disease. Jane faces ongoing personal torment as she struggles with love / hate feelings toward her husband. Attending a family support group could help Jane distinguish her love for her husband from her hatred for the disease that alters his behaviors.

This isn't the way it was supposed to be

Memory impairment steals away spouses, parents, grandparents, companions, and friends. Spouses who spent years planning to travel the country in their camper have to modify or give up those plans. Young adults are forced to become parents to their parents at a time in their lives when they thought that Mom or Dad would still be available for guidance and encouragement. Grandchildren lose the opportunities to spend the weekend or go fishing with grandparents. Elder companions who might have developed a lasting relationship, must move on or become a caregiver. Some senior adults have already performed years of caregiving for a mate who died. Their compassion level is too drained to begin that process again. Friends give up the interests they shared and gradually drift apart. Retirement planning is about fun, freedom, new faces and new places. No one makes advance plans for memory impairment. It merely happens to individuals, their families, and friends. Memory impairment is the camouflaged quicksand pit along the road to the golden years.

Economic Changes

An early stage diagnosis of memory impairment gives the family time to make appropriate financial and legal arrangements while the affected person can still participate in the planning. All too often, dementia is identified after the individual loses the capacity for decision making. Dealing with financial and legal matters at the later stages of memory impairment becomes increasingly complicated.

Protection of assets and income is crucial.

Forgetfulness and a struggle to appear in control leads some early stage memory impaired persons to make reckless decisions with money. Consider the frequent unsolicited mail order items or magazine subscriptions carefully disguised as bills. These are just some of the money schemes that prey on the elderly, particularly the confused elderly. Even legitimate charitable requests for money can be so touching that a person responds beyond reasonable means.

Evie remembers how hard life was growing up during the Great Depression. Anytime she sees a fund-raising letter with pictures of poorly clothed, sad-eyed children, she feels compelled to give money. Her previous approach was to budget a certain amount monthly for charitable giving and alternate between the charities. Over the past year as she became more forgetful, she wrote checks without balancing her checkbook. She does not understand that the money being drained from her savings to cover regular monthly checking overdrafts is rapidly dwindling.

Unless an alert bank officer sees the repeated overdraft notices and talks with Evie, the problem may not be discovered until it's too late to protect her savings. Her only son, who lives across the country, has respected his mother's privacy about money. By the time he visits again, Evie's funds may be depleted because of her generosity.

Set up a legal safety net

Evie needs an appropriate legal arrangement to avoid losing her income and assets due to irresponsible spending. At least that's one problem Jane does not have. As soon as Jane and Jacob retired, they set up a Living Trust with appropriate provisions so that either spouse could manage the finances if the other spouse died, became disabled, or incapacitated. The family or spouse of a newly diagnosed memory impaired person needs immediate legal counsel to review the options for financial management and estate planning. Look for an attorney and financial planner who is trained in elder law issues; trusts, asset protection, financing for long term care, and the assistance available for home or facility care through Medicare and Medicaid. Whether the family/couple decides to implement a Living Trust, Will, Health Care Surrogate, Durable Family Power of Attorney or Legal Guardianship depends on the overall financial situation and long term objectives.

Another valuable source of assistance to the family is a *case manager*. The case manager functions somewhat like the coach of a sports team; look over each situation, select the right "players," plan the moves and direct the action toward the goal. A case manager may be assigned to those who qualify through a public agency such as Medicaid. Case management services are also available on a fee for service basis from private companies. For families who live longer distances from a memory impaired relative, the case manager can be another important safety net. Consult the telephone directory, area Office of Aging, physicians, or the nearest Alzheimer's Association group to ask for recommendations of case management services.

Adjust to living on a reduced income

An ever increasing number of senior adults continue to work after their first retirement to supplement a meager or nonexistent pension. The onset of memory impairment that affects the working senior adult brings an additional financial burden for the family or couple. Often the result is a dramatic lifestyle change to reduce expenses. The nonimpaired spouse is hit with a double punch; facing loss of companionship plus moving to cheaper, less desirable housing and slashing the budget to bare bones existence.

The stress on the spouse to learn new caregiving duties, accept the reality of the disease, and make lifestyle changes that conform to the reduced income, pushes many stable people over the edge into depression. At this time, when so much attention is given to the memory impaired person, physicians and other professionals need to be sensitive to the depression, adjustment, and loss issues of the spouse as caregiver.

Estimate the costs of caregiving

Whether the memory impaired person lives at home, in an assisted living facility or a nursing home depends on the level of care needs and the availability of a person or persons to consistently provide those needs. Don't assume that home care is substantially less expensive than facility care until counting the full costs. The spouse or family must make estimates of annual expenses to develop a monthly budget. Consider these questions:

How will lost income be replaced?

What other investment income is available?

What financial planning needs to be implemented so that the cost of caring for the memory impaired person will not wipe out the savings and resources of the surviving spouse or family?

What public assistance is available?

Will additional medical supplies be needed such as hospital bed, shower chair, ramp, rails, wheelchair, walker or other equipment?

Is there a need for regular home health aides or visiting nurses? If yes, what is the cost? Will Medicare or other payors assist with the costs?

How much environmental remodeling must be done to make the home safe for a memory impaired person?

Are transportation services available that cater to the requirements of the infirm or wheelchair bound persons?

At what price?

Is there any financial assistance for transportation services?

What opportunities exist for adult daycare or respite care?

What is the cost of daycare or respite care?

Is transportation provided to the adult daycare?

What emergency backup system is in place to care for the memory impaired person if the caregiver becomes ill, injured, or hospitalized? Where? How much?

Who will coordinate the transfer of the memory impaired person to interim care?

Answering these questions guides the spouse and family in developing a caregiving action plan and an economic overview. If long term care in assisted living or a nursing home is an option, then compare the monthly fees of facility care with that of home care. Remember that there are personal costs for home caregiving which do not appear directly on a budget. A caregiver may begin with a firm resolve to keep the spouse or parent in the home. As the years go by and functioning declines, fewer of those people who said "call on me anytime" are available. The primary caregiver may need to re-examine the home care decision and consider facility care.

Activity Changes

Social life changes, but does not have to end

After retirement, Jane and Jacob couldn't get enough of playing bridge and golf with other couples. These activities became the core of their social life. They looked forward to the monthly dinners sponsored by the Tee for Two couples' golf group. After Jacob was diagnosed with Alzheimer's disease, the men in the golf group continued to try to include him in activities. They would invite him to join their practice sessions at the driving range. When Jacob could no longer safely swing a golf club, he was content to ride in the cart with Jane and another couple and watch them play golf.

Once Jacob's unpredictable anger outbursts began, Jane withdrew quietly from the bridge club and the couples golf group. She made excuses so often that the other couples thought she had lost interest in cards or golf. Her neighbor, Cora, knew the truth. She watched Jane's usually bright smile disintegrate into a wrinkled frown. Cora arrived one morning with fresh muffins and took over like a drill sergeant. She told Jane to get dressed while she prepared breakfast for Jacob. When Jane returned to the kitchen, Cora gave her a news clipping with the address of the local Memory Impairment Family Group's morning coffee meeting at nearby Community Church. She insisted on staying with Jacob so that Jane could attend the meeting.

Weeks later Jane said, "Cora's kindness saved my life. I thought the social life I so dearly looked forward to in retirement was over forever. The family group taught me how to arrange meaningful activities for me and for Jacob." Jane still plays golf, only she switched to a women's group that meets on Tuesday mornings while Jacob attends adult daycare. She found six spouses in the Memory Impairment Family Group who like to play bridge. These serious bridge players meet at the local Senior Center in a small card room. They have a rotating schedule; four spouses play cards while the other two conduct an informal activity group with the memory impaired persons in the Center's craft room. By reserving these rooms in an easily accessible recreational space with a built-in care option, there's fun for everyone. Jane and the other caregivers are able to socialize and take a break from their duties, knowing that the memory impaired spouses are safe and occupied.

Planning replaces spur-of-the-moment actions
Couples and families who enjoy the impromptu picnics and last minute decisions to drive to the fishing cabin for the weekend will have to learn in advance how to plan for the needs of the memory impaired person. For example, some types of vacations and family events can overwhelm the memory impaired person with excess stimulation and inadequate time for relaxation. As wonderful as trips can be, getting away from home usually means a change of routines. Breaking away from a consistent routine may be liberating for the caregiver but disorienting and fearful to the memory impaired person.

The free-wheeling, "don't-fence-me-in" type of families may find that long term caregiving simply does not work with their lifestyle. Those who cannot or will not adapt their leisure pursuits to a degree that is comfortable to the confused person definitely need to seek other caregiving options.

Separation of activities can benefit everyone
Jane and her friends from the family group discovered how well this separation of activities works for nonimpaired and impaired persons. Of the utmost importance is that the caregiver never has to feel guilty about planning separate activities. If the caregiver likes to attend concerts and the spouse can't sit still or quiet during a long performance, then the event becomes a disaster for both of them (and the audience nearby). Better to ask a relative or friend to visit and entertain the memory impaired person while the caregiver attends the concert. In another situation, a calm natured memory impaired person may enjoy drawing pictures with the children while the nonimpaired partner helps the neighbor do a woodworking project. As long as the memory impaired person is engaged in a safe activity within sight (or with supervision), the nonimpaired partner has more than earned the opportunity to enjoy time with friends.

Conduct a mental rehearsal before any social event or trip.
The best way to avoid an unpleasant response away from home is to consider the location, schedule, stressor and pleasures of the occasion. Just like athletes and other performers, caregivers can take a mental walk through the planned activity and imagine how to handle various possibilities. If the caregiver decides to bring her memory

impaired spouse to a formal concert, then they need to reserve seats on the aisle near an exit. Then if the confused person becomes agitated, they can easily leave with minimal disturbance to other people. Another option is to attend a matinee performance which may not be as crowded. The memory impaired person who likes to walk may be able to accompany a spouse to the shopping mall or grocery store. Again, go at the times and days that are less crowded. Definitely avoid lengthy shopping during holidays when overstimulation is at a height, shoppers are pushy, and tempers flare. During any outing, take ample sit-down breaks and be alert to nearest rest rooms. Some locations are just not suitable such as an outdoor flea market, the county fair or a discount store clearance sale. The noise, unstructured spaces and heightened activity are prime conditions for agitation, hallucinations and wandering.

Understand that a memory impaired person's interests can change.
As functioning abilities decline, a memory impaired person becomes easily frustrated with activities that were formerly pleasurable. One of Gaylene's longtime favorite ways to relax was watercolor painting. She often carried a small watercolor kit in her suitcase as she traveled during her modeling years. For the first year she lived in assisted care, she painted during expressive arts group. The art therapist noticed that Gaylene would start to paint, then stare at the paper finally bursting out in tears.

Because of memory loss, watercolor painting ceased to be relaxing and became disorienting and irritating. Although Gaylene would no longer hold a paint brush, she continued to stare at the arts group as if she felt like she no longer belonged. The art therapist bought some non-toxic, large color markers and a coloring book with simple pictures. She demonstrated how to use the markers. Gaylene can spend an hour coloring with the easy to hold markers. She seems to again find delight as the bright colors emerge on the paper. A considerate art therapist found a different way for Gaylene to connect with a life-long interest.

Spouse and family caregivers are often surprised when the memory impaired person suddenly rejects a favorite activity. Don't be. Expect change even though there's no indication of when that change is about to happen. Flexibility is important. Never try to persuade the confused person to resume an activity. If possible, like the art therapist did, find alternative ways to participate. A memory impaired person who liked dancing may one day refuse to dance with a spouse. Instead of dancing, sit together and listen to the music.

Location Changes

Leaving the family home is difficult.
Due to financial pressure or the decision to arrange care in a facility, the memory impaired person faces the added confusion of leaving familiar home surroundings. Making this move in the early stages of memory impairment is both easier and harder. It's easier in that the person has more functioning abilities to use in adjustment and socialization. The harder part is that the memory impaired person experiences a separation anxiety, a lingering sadness at leaving the spouse, family, and home.

Those persons who have the most difficult adjustment may not become settled in the new surroundings until reaching the next stage of cognitive decline. On the bright side, some memory impaired persons who seemed apathetic and irritable at home are revitalized from the increased activity and interaction with other seniors. There is no way to predict how the memory impaired person will respond.

The best way to support the adjustment is for spouse and family to show a positive attitude about the move. Save any concerns or doubts to discuss with a counselor, support group, or trusted friend.

One approach to making the transition is to bring the memory impaired person to the facility for a morning group or lunch (with prior facility approval) for several days before the move. Don't expect the confused person to learn how to get around the facility or totally understand the transition. However, even the brief exposures to the facility and residents makes it feel somewhat less alien to the newcomer.

Environmental changes are challenging for everyone
The changes within the home to accommodate a memory impaired person will be beneficial over the long term of caregiving. Remember that these changes also demand adaptation by the nonimpaired spouse and family members. Even subtle changes in furniture arrangement,

removing favorite (now unsafe) decorator objects and adding hall-way rails can appeal to the logical mind and upset the aesthetic sensibilities. Adult children and grandchildren may be the ones to complain most when the heirloom umbrella stand is removed from the hallway or they have to fight with safety latches to open the kitchen cabinents. The message is: "things aren't the way they use to be and that's hard to accept." For the memory impaired person, some changes in the environment are resisted while others are easily adaptable. These changes are ultimately designed for protection, ease of movement and to support independence for the memory impaired resident. As discussed in the chapter on modifying the environment, the caregiver and other family members can still have their favorite decor and breakables in their own locked rooms. Open access rooms must be rearranged to be as safe as possible.

Travel demands the simplest route between two points.
Right after retirement, Jane and Jacob took advantage of many travel opportunities. They bought 21-day train tickets and stopped in several cities on the way to visit relatives in California. Flying to New England to visit Jacob's sister, they would take an early flight with a long layover in Atlanta. Jane's childhood friend, Audrey Lee, met them at the airport for lunch. Jacob, who always liked to travel, now becomes agitated and confused on long trips. He can no longer participate in the pleasurable stopovers they used to share with friends like Audrey Lee.

Jane learned some valuable travel tips from the memory impairment support group. She looks for midweek nonstop flights in the evening. Jacob is more likely to fall asleep with the interior airplane lights dim and less noise from other sleepy passengers. Airport terminals are not as busy at night and midweek. Long trips to California or the Aruba resort they previously enjoyed are more than Jacob can manage. Even driving more than two hours to visit friends across the state is too confining for Jacob. So Jane asked these longtime friends to meet them halfway. They make lunch reservations at a quiet restaurant. On the way home, Jacob often takes a nap in the backseat.

Any travel, local or longer distances, needs to be broken down into small segments. Another option for a longer trip is to get settled into a motel in midafternoon. Take a walk for exercise. Have dinner in a quiet place or order room service. Start traveling again the next morning after the commuter rush.

Routines are usually upset when traveling. The lack of consistency and the overstimulation potential in busy transportation hubs can be disorienting and very stressful for the memory impaired person. At that point, the caregiver needs to travel after finding respite care in a facility or arranging in-home care for the resident. Both persons can have a more satisfying, restful time when travel options are viewed realistically rather than idealistically.

Relationships - Economics - Activities - Location: no matter how effectively or how poorly caregivers respond, these REAL changes seem to be the source of most distress among family members as the memory impairment progresses.

What happens next?

Family caregivers frequently ask how to recognize the characteristics of each stage in the progression of memory impairment. What can we expect next? When will the changes begin? What do we do? With all these uncertainties, families become highly frustrated because physicians, psychologists, nurses, social workers, home health aides, and other health care providers cannot give precise answers to their questions.

The behaviors and skill losses of memory impairment can occur at various times or stages of impairment. As a genuine effort to help caregivers recognize the disease progression, without offering absolutes, the following list of symptoms is presented. The order of stages is based on the Global Deterioration Scale previously introduced in Chapter 2. Memory impaired persons remain unique human beings and may not experience all of the characteristics noted in a given stage, or they may engage in certain behaviors during a different stage than other persons.

Stage 1: No notable memory problems

Any incidents of forgetfulness are part of the normal aging process and do not compromise social or occupational functioning.

Stage 2: Cognitive decline is very mild.

Forgetfulness is more frequent than in prior adult years, including: losing familiar objects like keys or wallet, forgetting names of friends, missing appointments, and being inconsistent with medication schedules.

A person is generally able to cover forgetfulness or mistakes on the job and in social situations.

Behavior changes may only be evident to spouse or family.

Any real problems are denied, yet the person may be fearful at onset of memory loss.

Performance on testing or in a clinical interview is usually adequate, thus diagnosis at this stage is rare.

Stage 3: Cognitive decline is mild.

Forgetfulness leads to confusion.

Losing objects is more frequent and lost items are more valuable (i.e., leaving a credit card at the store or becoming frustrated trying to find own car in a crowded parking lot).

There is risk of minor injury to self or others from household accidents (i.e., forgetting to clean up spilled water).

An inability to hide mistakes at work may result in losing a job or being forced to accept early retirement.

A newspaper story cannot be discussed shortly after reading it.

Self care reminders are occasionally needed.

Performance deficits on testing and in clinical interview may be sufficient to detect memory loss.

Stage 4: Cognitive decline is moderate

Forgetfulness and confusion is frequent and significant.

Well known places are usually easily navigated, but confusion results from multi-step directions.

There is some loss or difficulty accessing long term memories. Short term memory is increasingly limited.

Forgetting names of some members of extended family is common, i.e., knows names of children and grandchildren, but not the names of their spouses or the great-grandchildren.

Person forgets to pay regular bills or pays inaccurate amount. The resulting delay in payments may result in cancellation of important items, such as electricity, medical supplement insurance, or other services.

His/her checkbook is not balanced. He or she cannot account for cash.

Orientation to time and place is periodically lost.

Hobbies or activities that involve complex instructions or abstract thinking, such as woodworking, sewing, computer, car repair, chess, or bridge club are given up.

The person uses denial as a cover-up for fear and confusion.

Some assistance with activities of daily living is needed.

He/she usually objects to the need for testing or evaluation.

Performance deficits on testing and in clinical interview are usually sufficient to detect memory loss.

Stage 5: Cognitive decline is moderately severe.

Living alone is no longer possible.

The person cannot perform all activities of daily living without prompting and/or assistance.

The person is capable of toileting and eating, but requires monitoring and some prompting.

Forgetfulness and confusion is chronic and distressing to the individual.

He/she cannot find the way around well known places without some assistance.

Names of some members of the family; grandchildren and extended family are forgotten. Information of recent births, marriages, or deaths in the family is not assimilated.

It is no longer safe to travel alone, even around a familiar neighborhood or town.

Talking about memories of self and family is common.

Certain stories are repeated frequently.

There is notable difficulty accessing short term memories.

The individual needs occasional reality orientation as to day, date, time, location, and season.

Performance deficits on testing and in clinical interview are sufficient to diagnose memory impairment.

Stage 6: Cognitive decline is severe.

Assistance with all activities of daily living is needed; the person may become incontinent.

The individual may wander away from home. For safety reasons, he/she requires round-the-clock monitoring or relocation to a secured living area.

He/she occasionally forgets the name of spouse or primary caregiver; typically does not recognize or understand the relationship of extended family, children, and grandchildren.

Short term memory is minimal.

Some long term memories remain, but may be limited to a few stories that are repeated frequently.

Reality orientation is vague. Generally, the person does not know the day, date, time, location, or season.

The person repeats one or two questions many times, which is frustrating to caregivers.

Increased frequency of problem behaviors is apparent.

By internal or external (environmental) triggers, he or she easily becomes delusional, disoriented, or obsessive.

Sleep patterns are disturbed. The person often wakes up in the late night hours and expects to begin daytime activities.

Loss of willpower and self directed action results.

Performance deficits on testing and in clinical interview are sufficient to diagnose memory impairment.

Stage 7: Cognitive decline is very severe.

Total care for activities of daily living is required.

Loss of meaningful verbal communication with only sounds of grunting or moaning is common.

Complete incontinence is experienced.

The person cannot walk or sit erect under his or her own power and must be moved regularly to prevent pressure sores.

The person needs help with feeding and drinking. Food choices are limited to what is easy to swallow and digest.

Basic directions cannot be followed.

The person does not recognize spouse, family or caregivers.

When Family Caregivers Yield to Professional Caregivers

Even the most dedicated family caregivers will turn to outside assistance for partial or total care if the disease progression is rapid or lengthy. The demands of being on-call 24 hours daily, week after week with only an hour or two of rest, result in physical and emotional exhaustion for many caregivers. For some caregivers, this collapse is a blessing in disguise because it takes a difficult decision out of the spouse's hands and prompts the family to act for him or her. Grandma may not be able to admit that she can no longer manage Grandpa. But if Grandma gets sick and the adult children relocate Grandpa to an assisted living facility, then she can passively accept the decision she refused to make on her own.

Other families take a more direct and realistic view of memory impairment. They understand that their caregiving potential is limited and so they explore alternative care options for the future. If the adult children honestly can't help with caregiving due to work schedules, raising small children or living too far away, then they can encourage the caregiver to be fair to himself or herself with regular breaks and mini-vacations.

One method of assessing the impact of caregiving on spouse and family is the Zarit Burden Interview. Answering these questions may help to get a realistic picture of the caregiver's feelings and whether or not to continue home care.

Ask the primary family caregiver to respond to these questions on the Zarit Burden Interview

1. Do you feel that your relative asks for more help than s/he needs?

2. Do you feel that because of the time you spend with your relative that you don't have enough time for yourself?

3. Do you feel stressed between caring for your relative and trying to meet other responsibilities for your family or work?

4. Do you feel embarrassed over your relative's behavior?

5. Do you feel angry when you are around your relative?

6. Do you feel that your relative currently affects your relationship with other family members or friends in a negative way?

7. Are you afraid what the future holds for your relative?

8. Do you feel your relative is dependent on you?

9. Do you feel strained when you are around your relative?

10. Do you feel your health has suffered because of your involvement with your relative?

11. Do you feel that you don't have as much privacy as you would like because of your relative?

12. Do you feel that your social life has suffered because you are caring for your relative?

13. Do you feel uncomfortable about having friends over because of your relative?

Zarit, S.H., Orr, N.K., & Zarit, J.M. (1985). *The hidden victims of Alzheimer's disease: families under stress.* New York University Press. Used with permission.

When the burden on the primary home caregiver becomes too great, that is the time to seek an appropriate level of assisted care for the memory impaired person. Although this is a difficult decision, the realistic family is totally supportive. Rather than moan, "it's so sad that Mom could no longer care for Dad," the supportive family says, "we so appreciate how much Mom did to care for Dad and now he needs another level of care." The way the family talks about the change in caregiving speaks volumes about how they really feel. To borrow an old-fashioned saying, "if the family can't say something positive about the home caregiver's efforts, then say nothing at all." The primary caregiver will feel both sad and relieved as the memory impaired person leaves home for facility care. This conflicting emotional tug is enough to handle without hearing indirect condemnation in the words of the family.

After the memory impaired person moves into the facility, the home caregiver must begin a new routine. Schedules change. Environmental adjustments (i.e., cabinet locks, signs, etc.) around the home can be removed. During this bittersweet time, some spouses are confused about making changes in the home. They have questions and thoughts that they are reluctant to relate to other family members:

"Is it wrong to pack up my wife's personal items as if she were dead?"

"What will my daughters think if I move into their old room and turn the master bedroom into a den?"

"If I take down the rails and ramp, am I admitting that my spouse will never come home again? Is that disloyal to the memories of our marriage?"

"My children are mad that I put the house up for sale the day after taking my wife to a nursing home. It wasn't reactive; I've thought about it for months. I'm sorry, but I just can't live here anymore. Without her, this house is a tomb for me."

Spouse or family caregivers need to be careful about acting hastily in any home or lifestyle decisions during this new grieving time. Many caregivers reach the decision for facility care out of desperation and exhaustion. Thus they have not allowed themselves to think about how to live the rest of their lives when full time caregiving duties are finished. For many caregivers, to plan ahead was the same as admitting that memory impairment has stolen their future with their spouse or parent. They heard the doctors say "no improvement is possible" and "this is a disease of progressively declining skills," but they could not focus on those predictions and still manage the day-to-day caregiving without hope. For those caregivers, yielding their loved ones to facility care is to abandon hope and deal with the harsh realities of the disease.

These changes are difficult even under the best of circumstances. During this process, the caregiver needs to be surrounded by caring family and friends, to participate in a support group and consider individual counseling by a professional familiar with the family issues of memory impairment. How effectively the caregiver resolves this transition period determines how productive and satisfying his or her remaining years will be. Failure to move on in life is to let the disease of dementia conquer two lives; the victim of the disease and the caregiver. There really is life after caregiving. Find a good support group or contact the Alzheimer's Association. From these sources, caregivers can meet others who have been where they are and found renewed meaning to life.

9

Stress: the Caregiver's Constant Companion

Identify the types of stress

Recognize sources of stress for family and staff caregivers

Ways to cope with stress

Stress from the Caregiver's Viewpoint

Elena, Tyronne and Cal are very different people who have arrived at their present locations through similar paths. They are in the later stages of memory impairment. In each situation, a spouse or family member started as primary home caregiver. As the disease progressed and the demands of caregiving steadily increased, each family reached the decision to bring their loved one to facility care.

Esteban barely knew how to use the kitchen appliances when Elena's functioning began to decline noticeably. The home was always her domain. She loved being a homemaker and mother. Then she declined to the point that she could not finish basic household tasks. Esteban didn't mind getting dishpan hands, trying to cook, or helping Elena bathe and dress. He was willing to do anything to keep Elena at home. His resolve was finally broken after Elena's angry outbursts and hallucinations overwhelming.

Their youngest daughter, Anna, returned from a teaching assignment in Peru and immediately became aware of the changes that memory impairment brought to her parents' lives. Anna couldn't decide whether she was more shocked by her mother's erratic behaviors or her father's extreme weight loss, sunken eyes, and exhaustion. She telephoned the other sisters to report what was happening. Then she learned that Elena's physician had recommended facility care months earlier. With support from her sisters, Anna persuaded Esteban to make the choice of a nursing home for Elena.

Tyronne became so forgetful in his duplex that he caused a kitchen fire. Fortunately, damage was moderate and no one was hurt. After that, Tyronne moved in with his son's family. Shandra, his daughter-in-law, became the primary caregiver with some assistance from her aunt who lived in the garage apartment. For a year, Shandra managed very well. With help from Aunt Minnie and friends from her church choir, Shandra had enough people to help with Tyronne so that she could take a break and continue volunteering with the Booster Club at her son's school.

"Almost overnight, Tyronne changed from a cooperative yet forgetful person to a verbally abusive tyrant," Shandra recalled. He began to push and curse at Shandra when she tried to help him dress. Yet when T.J. came home, Tyronne was a different person. T.J. didn't see as much of the erratic behaviors that were so stressful to Shandra and Aunt Minnie.

Finally Tyronne's paranoia increased to the point that he began telling people at church and in the neighborhood that Shandra was trying to poison him. T.J. did not realize how difficult this problem was until he got a frantic phone call from the city jail. Apparently someone took Tyronne's paranoid rambling seriously and made a report of "elder abuse" against Shandra. T.J. rushed to the jail. He called the family physician to talk with the police investigator. The physician verified Tyronne's memory impairment and his unusual behaviors just as Shandra tried to tell the officers. As T.J. escorted his wife to the car, he knew this was a turning point. Shandra's voice was shaking as she quietly said, "I've done my best with Tyronne but I can't do this anymore. T.J., you must choose who remains at home either him or me, but not both of us." The next day they began looking for a nearby assisted care facility. Three days later, Tyronne was moved to City Nursing Center. Shandra faithfully visited, often on her way to counseling. Several months of psychotherapy were needed for Shandra to overcome the trauma of being arrested and her feelings of failure for not being able to continue caregiving.

According to Bonnie, Cal had "low blood sugar that made him forgetful." She was so good at covering up his memory impairment that their daughter, Cally, did not realize the truth of Cal's condition. Bonnie refused to believe the diagnosis of Alzheimer's disease. She was committed to taking care of Cal at home.

Cal never understood why Bonnie didn't come home anymore. Cally tried to explain that Bonnie had a sudden heart attack while sweeping the patio. Cal does not remember the neighbor rushing over to help or the paramedics arriving with the ambulance. He just knows that Bonnie "went somewhere." Within one day, Cally, a single mother of two, had to cope with the death of her mother and a new awareness of her father's dementia.

Rather than uproot her children and move back home, Cally arranged for Cal's widowed sister, Claire, to be a live-in caregiver. Cally telephoned frequently and packed the children in the car driving ten hours round trip to visit every two weeks. Her visits gave Claire a weekend off duty. After eight months, Claire was so nervous and exhausted that she refused to stay. Cally's only remaining choice was assisted care, yet she felt guilty that Cal could not remain at home as her mother wanted.

Cally thought that moving Dad into the facility would be awful. At the intake meeting, the social worker introduced them to Joanne, a patient care aide on the unit where Cal was assigned. Joanne recognized Cally's distress and Cal's fears. She was calm, reassuring and cheerful. Cal seemed to like her. Joanne wrote down Cally's address and promised to help Cal write letters to the grandchildren. Cally never imagined finding such a compassionate paid caregiver as Joanne. Over time, Cally marveled at how special Joanne was. In her heart she knew that Bonnie would have approved of how Joanne cared for Cal.

Joanne has been a patient care aide for nine years. During that time, she worked in a hospital and several nursing homes. She finds the daily tasks routine and manageable. Joanne has learned from other staff members and additional in-service training how to deal with the difficult behaviors and unexpected actions of memory impaired persons. Her greatest challenges come from dealing with some staff and family members.

After years of experience, Joanne still gets upset when other staff caregivers are lazy, complaining and ignoring resident requests. She dreads being second-guessed by family members who spend more time criticizing the staff than visiting with their relative. As the resident's functioning declines, some family members try to blame the caregivers.

She wishes that outsiders would realize how the staff and residents become a "family" over years together. As she gently washes Cal's face, she remembers how active he was when he arrived. She enjoyed playing the guitar as he sang old cowboy songs. Now he cannot speak or respond. Joanne has been there day after day to witness the decline to this final stage of dementia. Cal's death is close. Cally calls daily to ask about her dad and to thank Joanne. That gratitude means more than Cally knows.

Sometimes Joanne wishes that she worked in a baby nursery where life begins instead of at a nursing home where life ends. Her Caring Caregivers Group talked about that at the last meeting. One of the advantages of working at a progressive facility like We Care Village is the availability of these groups for the staff. Each group is small, limited to a maximum of ten caregivers. There are dozens of similar groups for staff on various shifts. At Caring Caregivers Group, Joanne and her colleagues talk about their feelings, discuss frustrations and learn about stress management. Joanne's job is both difficult and rewarding. Since she began participating in the Caring Caregivers Group, Joanne is managing her stress at work and home much better.

Recognizing Stress

Stress is a real concern, whether the caregiver is on duty for eight hour shifts in a nursing home or on 24 hour call as a home caregiver. Meeting the needs of the most frail and impaired persons is at the heart of caregiver stress. Add marriage conflicts, problems with children, lack of sleep, financial worries, and other real life concerns to this anticipated work related stress and the caregiver is overwhelmed.

An overly stressed caregiver is less effective and less alert to needs or dangers.

Like Joanne, many paid caregivers are prepared to deal with the demands of resident care but are easily blind-sided by staff, administration, and families. A facility caregiver is affected by an overly critical supervisor, being denied a pay increase, reassignment to a new unit, or waiting for the state inspection team to arrive.

Home caregivers, like Shandra, are affected by dramatic changes in family routine, losing contact with friends, lack of appreciation, and feeling like a failure. Compound those concerns with other stressors such as holiday preparations, inadequate time to spend with the children, giving up social or volunteer pursuits, and loss of intimacy with one's spouse due to caregiving demands.

The first step toward dealing with stress is to recognize the sources of stress in the caregiver's life. Some can be changed and others cannot. However, all stress can be managed once it is identified and acknowledged.

Different Types of Stress

All humans experience stress. A "stress-free life" is impossible. Feeling stress is not the problem. Trying to avoid stress is not the answer. What a person does with stress is a much greater problem than the existence of stress.

Stress is merely a demand oriented response with notable physical and emotional arousal.

Stress is an equal opportunity problem, moving across the lines of gender, race, economics, and location. Examples are easy to find. Surgical trauma teams are capable of channeling their skills and attention to respond to the demands of saving lives. A college student insists that his best work is done when facing a deadline on a term paper. The surgical team and the college student are responding to their stresses in a productive manner. Highly successful Wall Street stockbrokers make or lose millions in a split second decision to sell a stock which may be productive stress for some stockbrokers and harmful stress to others. A premature infant struggles for breath as her parents watch helplessly. A department store manager is laid off from work with less than a year until expected retirement. The stress of that infant's parents and the department store manager are harmful stresses.

Stress is either "harmful" or "productive"

Harmful stress is negative, painful, sad, oppressive, and overwhelming. The by-products of harmful stress are anxiety, depression, substance abuse, high blood pressure, becoming accident prone, and psychosomatic illness. This type of stress may result in physical symptoms that command immediate attention for survival. Over time, harmful stress causes the worst kind of wear and tear on the human body and a weight to the human spirit. No wonder some people who are overcome by harmful stress try to numb their pain with alcohol, drugs, food, shopping, gambling, or other addictive behaviors.

Not all stress is harmful. The human body also reacts to productive stress like the anticipation of a special event, anxiously awaiting a loved one to arrive at the airport, or pushing past previous endurance in running a race. By its very nature, productive stress gives a person the extra drive to produce something new, faster, better or more creatively. An actor can feel stress before the curtain goes up yet give a fantastic performance. The actor's productive stress becomes part of the acting process and is used to energize the outcome. For many people, stress is harmful and negatively impacts the outcome. Learning to distinguish and redirect the power of stress is very important for caregivers.

Major Stressors for Facility Caregivers

Repetitive duties
The essential resident care tasks such as bathing, dressing, toileting, feeding, and encouraging appropriate activity never change. Day after day these routine jobs take up a substantial part of the workload for patient care aides, CNA's and other direct service providers.

Coping with difficult behaviors
In a single day, a facility caregiver encounters all the of the difficult behaviors discussed in a previous chapter. Any one behavioral problem can be tiring to handle. Multiply that by twenty residents for eight hours a day, and the caregiver's compassion is rapidly drained.

Inadequate training in working with the memory impaired

Training for nurses aides, CNAs, and other support staff is usually general and task related. It's the exceptional program that teaches the special issues and needs of a person with memory impairment. Even the simple understanding that cursing, hitting, and biting are just manifestations of the disease, not the resident's choice, helps caregivers cope with the work better.

Lack of cooperation from coworkers

Many caregiving tasks take two persons; such as bathing a reluctant or frail resident. When one worker tries to dump the less desirable duties on another worker, stress levels and tempers escalate. Memory impaired residents may not understand the problem, but they often react to the anxiety and anger that emanates from caregivers.

Demanding supervisor

A critical, perfectionist or blaming supervisor adds a stress load to the caregiver that is far greater than any difficult resident behavior. Memory impaired persons don't realize the impact of their actions. A demanding supervisor has no excuse for acting with poor management style, insensitivity, and over-control.

Status more important than team approach

Health care, like many fields, has a status structure based on education and professional license. The people at the highest level of skills may perform the more desirable duties while those at the lower levels of training perform the repetitive, less desirable duties. The line of "status" is an arbitrary divider that creates a destructive "them" and "us" division. In a team approach, every caregiver has specific duties. However, no one is above helping, encouraging or lending support as needed to any other team member. A team approach is clearly in the best interest of staff and residents.

Limited opportunities for promotion or pay increase

The hardest working direct service providers are on the lower levels of pay. Real career advancement is not likely without additional education or license. Caregivers at the aide level are often on hourly pay with erratic shift schedules and fewer employee benefits. Job security is non-existent.

Major Stressors for Family Caregivers

Repetitive duties
The primary home caregiver becomes responsible for the essential tasks of bathing, dressing, toileting, feeding, and encouraging appropriate activity for the memory impaired person. A family caregiver must become aware of anticipating these needs for a person who was independent for so many years. These routine yet necessary care duties consume a large portion of the caregiver's day and further isolate the caregiver from contact with other people in work or leisure activities.

Coping with difficult behaviors
The family caregiver must deal with a range of difficult and changeable behaviors just like a facility caregiver. However, the family caregiver has the added emotional burden of watching a loved one suddenly act hostile, paranoid, aggressive, or fearful. The emotional burden on the family caregiver is very high.

Inadequate training about memory impairment
A typical family caregiver knows almost nothing about memory impairment until this disease strikes someone in their home. The family caregiver is usually thrust into this role by demand or default with no preparation in basic aide work, the progression of memory impairment, or essential behavior management techniques. Attending family support groups and reading as much as possible about memory impairment helps family caregivers survive the on-job-training.

Lack of support from family and community
Facility caregivers may have lazy coworkers, but at least there are other persons to lend a hand. A family caregiver may spend all or most of every day alone with the memory impaired person. The family caregiver can't even take a shower without first making certain that the memory impaired person is safe and secure. The strain of being on duty 24 hours, seven days weekly is too much for anyone. Without some regular periods of time off (a few hours to a few days) the family caregiver will suffer physical or emotional breakdown. Ask for help. Ask other family members to sit with the resident while the caregiver attends church, shops, or goes to lunch with friends. When necessary, find adult daycare or facilities with respite care programs.

Role conflicts

Family caregivers frequently report the greatest difficulties when the resident is a parent or in-law. The conditioning is strong: parents make decisions and children follow their parents' lead. Memory impairment changes those relationships. Now the adult child is the parent to the parent. The family caregiver worries about being too bossy or causing the older person to feel demeaned when frequent reminders are needed for even basic tasks.

Role confusion

Spouse caregivers feel tremendous inner conflict at becoming the parent to their partner. The balance of the marriage is upset by the changing roles. Other family caregivers feel the conflicts as well. Some wonder if they are giving the proper respect to the elder whose diapers they change. The patriarch or matriarch of the family spends more time coloring with the grandchildren than being with the adults. Adjusting to the changes brought on by the disease process is challenging for everyone.

Limited opportunities for personal time

Family caregivers easily become so over-tired from tending to the activities of daily living, that they isolate from the rest of the world. They become so captive to being "on call" that they forget their own needs for relaxation. The home is no longer an oasis of comfort and solace, it's a workplace.

Stress Response Mistakes

As previously stated, stress is not the problem. How people respond to stress is where problems begin. The worst possible caregiver responses to stress are seen in the following caregiver personalities.

The General seeks to conquer the caregiving problems with an aggressive stand. Use whatever is necessary to achieve the goal: demanding, shouting, demeaning, or just moving the resident. If the resident balks, show a superior attitude until the objective is achieved.

The Boxer pulls no punches to fight combativeness with greater force. Rather than get out of the way of a flailing resident, grab their arms and prove who is stronger. Forget that the resident under attack is less likely to calm down or diminish combativeness simply by being subdued.

The Blamer holds the memory impaired resident responsible for erratic behaviors, instead of the disease. Always on the defensive, the Blamer never accepts any responsibility for helping the resident function within the environment. In a facility, the Blamer points the finger toward another staff member as the cause of the problem.

The Martyr is long suffering in a thankless job and wants everyone to know about it. In reciting a litany of problems that make up the daily schedule, the Martyr wears out the patience of family and friends who might otherwise lend a hand. In a facility, the Martyr takes the tough jobs then complains bitterly about being poorly treated by co-workers and the supervisor.

The Philosopher gets side-tracked looking for some deeper meaning to the memory impairment. Is this a punishment for hidden misdeeds? Will this disease become a family curse? Are safety restrictions for the memory impaired person a way to limit free expression? It is amazing how philosophy can become a way to avoid reality and deny stress by twisting it into an intellectual exercise.

The Ostrich is passively trying to get by each day. Under the guise of not being controlling, the Ostrich secretly hopes that inaction will motivate someone else to act. If the memory impaired person acts up during an over stimulating family gathering, then maybe someone else will take charge. That way the Ostrich does not have to appear weak in asking for help or be the one to make the decision. In a facility, the Ostrich staff member tries not to see a resident in need or hear a call from the bathroom. By creating busy work at the chart file, the Ostrich simply can't leave the chosen task to do the less desirable job.

Developing Coping Skills

Stressful people, places, or jobs that cannot be changed or ignored must be managed with coping skills that are used to defuse stress responses. Notice how some people can stay "cool and calm" in the midst of a stressful situation while other people are anxious and frantic. If the situation is the same, what makes the difference? Coping skills make the difference. In all levels of health care, dealing with people who are sick, dependent and needy, coping skills are essential to continue in this work. Coping skills are just as important for family caregivers, who may never have had the opportunity for this type of training.

Stress Inoculation Method

Meichenbaum and Cameron (1974) created a method called "stress inoculation" to teach better ways of responding to stress. Using this method, a caregiver would plan and write down several short statements that apply to the four key phases of dealing with stress:

1. Preparing to encounter stress,

2. Facing a stressful situation,

3. Admitting fears about the situation, and

4. Verbally rewarding a successful response.

Applying this method to a stressful situation with a memory impaired person might include statements such as these:

"Cursing is just a sign that Harry is upset." (Prepare for the stress)
"If I slow down and talk to Harry, he won't need to curse to get attention." (Face the stressful situation)

"Even if he curses, he doesn't do it to demean me or frighten me." (Admit fears)

"When I take more time talking with Harry, I can help him to settle down and be more cooperative about dressing." (Verbally reinforce or praise success)

Identify at least four caregiving situations that continually represent stress in the home or facility. Apply the "stress inoculation" method to each situation. If you are part of a caregiver support group or at staff meetings, try to think of alternative ways to respond to stress. Write the statements chosen for each situation on 3x5 index cards that fit easily into pocket or purse. Carry these cards and review frequently. After some practice and successful responses, this coping skill will become easier and easier to follow.

The stress inoculation response is one method that gives the caregiver a renewed feeling of strength in coping with the difficult and unpredictable behaviors of the memory impaired.

Stress Priority List

All stressful situations are not equal. If stress were a number, it's value would vary according to each person's perception. For paramedics, the sight of blood on an injured person in a traffic accident is not particularly stressful. A bystander who has never seen such a serious injury could feel highly stressed over witnessing the same scene. The situation is the same, but stress level is different depending on the viewpoint of each individual.

Family and facility caregivers are subject to the same type of stresses in caring for the memory impaired. The question for each caregiver to answer is "what types of stress are most difficult for me?" This process is quite simple. Take a piece of paper and write or type a list of the most stressful activities of caregiving. Be specific. Avoid writing an overly broad item such as, "lunch time." Instead, consider what it is about lunch time that is stressful. Potential lunch time stresses are: getting the resident to remain seated, serving food, wiping up spills, responding to swallowing distress, or encouraging the resident to eat.

In making the stress list also note stresses that belong to the caregiver such as, "rushing through my lunch," "a co-worker who won't do certain cleaning if it messes up her manicure," or "feeling unappreciated for my efforts."

After completing the list, rank each item by the letters, A,B,C. "A" stresses are major concerns that can really ruin the day. "B" stresses are important concerns that can be managed with some effort. "C" stresses are irritating and unpleasant, but not enough to ruin the day. When time permits, rewrite the list by grouping together all A's, B's, and C's. Which category has the most items? If it's "A," are you sure that all these stresses are really "A list" events? Could you be looking at too many things in life as dreadful, impossible or devastating? If yes, reorder the list again.

The stress priority list suggests what areas need immediate attention to reduce caregiver stress. Sometimes just seeing on paper these concerns that bounce around the brain like popcorn popping helps to bring order to mental chaos. The caregiver may want to apply the stress inoculation method to each stress item. Eliminate as many "C" list items as possible to prove you can do it, then move on the "A" list or tackle one item at a time from the "A" list then work your way down to "B" and "C." Any problem solving is more effective if it is consistent with the caregiver's personality and overall approach to other life decisions.

Simple Relaxation Exercises

Does the idea of relaxation amid the many caregiving duties seem ridiculous? Actually, relaxation for caregivers is a sanity saver that is well worth the few minutes it takes. Here are a few simple exercises for busy caregivers:

Personal motivation

Prepare one or two brief statements that act as your personal motivation in any situation. For a caregiver that might be: "This anger isn't directed at me, it's the disease." Substitute any problem behavior where "anger" appears in the statement. Another personal motivation is: "I trust my ability to handle _____." Fill in that blank as needed. "I trust my ability to handle this resident's paranoia." When you feel tension, repeat your personal motivation as frequently as needed.

Counting blessings

Instead of reviewing the frustrations over your coffee break, count the blessings that you have seen. Count everything. Nothing is too small or too insignificant. For example, "Mrs. Smith took a shower with only a few words of complaint. There was a good parking spot open this morning. Taking a resident out for a walk gave me time to enjoy being outside." When taking a break, really break away from the stresses by focusing attention on positive thoughts.

Take a real breather

Get away from the place where tension began. Step outside the room door, onto the porch or into the bathroom. Take in deep, lung filling breaths and slowly exhale. Focus attention on inhaling and exhaling. Notice your body begin to relax and let go of that tension. Deep breathing is the opposite of the shallow, panting breathing that accompanies stress.

Enjoy a walking break

Who says that a coffee break must be spent sitting and drinking caffeine? Use break time to walk around the block or the parking lot. Bring bottled water along to drink during a brisk walk. Or have a slow walk for meditation and spiritual reflection. Think about who you are and what you contribute to your corner of the world.

Make a picture escape

Bring a photo of a wonderful vacation or a travel brochure of the vacation spot of your dreams. During a break, look at that photo. Recall pleasant times past or weave a fantasy. As you look deeply at the photo, use all your senses. Identify in detail the sounds, smells, and tastes. Was there warm sand under your feet or flakes of new fallen snow? Paint a rich view with as much related information as possible. That's your fifteen minute vacation escape using a beautiful picture to stimulate a short, satisfying relaxation experience.

Healthy Responses to Stress

Caregivers must learn how to care for themselves in order to be effective in caring for others. Developing and regularly practicing a good self-care regime is important for family caregivers and facility caregivers. Here's how to begin new healthy responses to stress:

Adequate nutrition

Essential to fuel the body for caregiving duties, getting enough of the right foods and vitamins also creates more alertness. Stress drains a lot of energy from the body. Replenish nourishment at regular intervals to boost energy levels.

Divide big jobs in manageable tasks

Looking at the entire day of caregiving duties can be staggering. At times, just getting a reluctant resident dressed is a big job. Break down that job into smaller parts. Start by talking to the resident and putting out clothing together. Take a short rest. Then begin to dress. If this does not work, go about another task as the resident calms. Perhaps there is no need to insist that slippers be replaced by shoes. The sturdy shoes can be put on later in the day when going outside. Divide the work to conquer the task with less distress on everyone involved.

Work with, not against, the body clock

Morning people are best on early shifts and evening people work well at night. As much as possible, sign up for shifts at times that match the body clock. For family caregivers, adjust some care tasks to productive times. An evening person may prefer to tackle difficult tasks with a resident such as bathing or hair washing in the later afternoon or early evening when the caregiver has more energy and patience.

Recognize limitations

One person can only do so much in a given time. When the duties of homemaking or mothering are compounded with caregiving for a memory impaired person, not everything on the "to do" list will happen. Prioritize tasks. Make schedules. In a facility, the caregiver must choose the essential tasks and follow procedures. As much as the caregiver wants to help a resident rearrange bureau drawers, that may need to wait until tomorrow so the most important care tasks are done on time.

Ask for help

As the months and years go by, other family and friends get busy with their lives and forget (or get tired of) the home caregiver's needs. Remind them that help is needed and offer specific choices of how to help ("will you sit with Grandpa on Tuesday during my appointment or fix dinner for him on Sunday while I'm at choir practice?").

Facility caregivers who are not getting cooperation from coworkers or whose workload is oppressive need to calmly state their concern to the appropriate supervisor. The issue is not that the caregiver is overworked. Instead, explain how an over-scheduled caregiver is not able to meet the resident needs and thus the residents are not getting what they need.

Find a safe place to vent emotions

A support group, a trusted friend, or a professional counselor are options for letting emotions be heard rather than bottled up. Caregivers remain healthier and more capable in performing their duties if they learn to accept their conflicting emotions as part of the role. Trying to deny conflicting emotions and personal distress is a quick road to serious physical and emotional problems.

Avoid blame

Casting blame is likely to reel in a whale of a lot of other problems. When attention is directed at finding someone to blame, the focus becomes firmly fixed on what is "wrong" rather that searching for ways to solve problems. Blaming is very energy depleting because it's so negative. That negative aspect of stress is physically harmful. Deal with the "facts" and stop wasting time on determining who or what could be at "fault." Learning to let go of blame is important in developing healthy responses to stress.

Exercise for enjoyment

This is important to let the body unwind. Find an activity that is fun either alone or with a group. Aerobics, running, and biking are great if done for fun. Forget competition. Walking and swimming are fine too. This is about helping the body relax by movement.

Make time for leisure pursuits

As strange as this sounds, caregivers usually have to schedule their leisure. Spur of the moment activities conflict with the consistency that a memory impaired person needs. Set a weekly appointment for time away from caregiving duties.

A family caregiver who feels isolated at home with a memory impaired person needs leisure plans that include socialization. Consider sports like tennis, golf, aerobics, or hiking with a group. Other less physical options are bridge, hobby groups, and special interest clubs.

The facility caregiver may feel overcome with responding to many people in a given day. Perhaps the best leisure choices are quiet activities that can be done alone or with others such as painting, crafts, sewing, gardening, biking, or photography.

REMEMBER: Stress is part of everyday life. For caregivers, the sources of stress are fairly predictable. Learning to recognize and respond to the stressors in healthy ways is the process known by the most effective family and facility caregivers.

10

When Caregiving Staff Become Wellness Facilitators

Developing a new view of caregiving

Recognize the impact of dependency and learned helplessness

Promote positive treatment objectives that focus on abilities rather than disabilities

Beliefs About Caregiving

Caregivers who work with the memory impaired need to examine their beliefs about this disease in a personal, not medical, manner. This is part of an important attitude adjustment that is the prelude to effective, sensitive, and respectful caregiving.

Let's begin with the basic principle of psychology, "behavior follows beliefs." Here's a simple illustration. Think of a person who has been told by a physician to stop drinking alcohol or face major physical complications. Faced with a grim prognosis and plenty of pressure from the family, the person successfully completes an alcohol treatment program and attends a support group twice weekly. There is a notable improvement in physical health. Changes in the person's work performance and overall temperament are clearly notable. From every outward appearance, the treatment is working. A few weeks later, the person begins sneaking alcohol and harmful physical symptoms resume. Why didn't the positive changes last? Simple. The underlying beliefs about alcohol and health never changed, therefore, the positive behavior change was not supported by the internal belief system.

This example shows the importance of changing negative beliefs in order to fully act on new, positive beliefs. Meaningful changes in approaches to caregiving begin with the caregiver. Without a real change of heart about caring for memory impaired persons, the techniques presented in this book will never be meaningful to the caregiver. Anything less than a change of beliefs about caregiving is just to go through the motions while the supervisor is watching only to return to mechanical, depersonalized approaches hours or days later.

Moving Beyond Caregiving

Caregiving in its traditional "caretaking" form or in less restrictive, more supportive models has emerged in the more enlightened model of "facilitating wellness." Rather than deal with the problems, behaviors and physical needs of the memory impaired as duties to scratch off a list, the concept of facilitating wellness is to assist where needed in preserving the independence and individuality of a memory impaired person. That's facilitating the resident's wellness.

A building block of facilitating wellness is in acquiring the knowledge and sensitivity necessary to reject "ageism." Just as racism is demeaning to persons of color, ageism is demeaning to older adults of all races, ethnicity, and cultures. Kermis (1984) wrote of the dangers of the "new ageism" as a second wave of discrimination by caregivers who have a negative attitude about elder patients. Kermis scolded health care workers at all levels from treating elders as a "waste of time" due to limited life spans and decreasing mental capacities. Ageism is more than telling rude jokes about aging or treating memory impaired persons in childlike ways. Ageism is any prejudice or stereotype that is applied to people because of age (Butler, Lewis, & Sunderland, 1991). A significant reason why depression is often ignored or untreated in older adults is because of the ageism in attitudes of physicians and other health care professionals (Katona, 1993).

Facilitating wellness means having as much concern about the emotional well-being of the memory impaired as about basic bodily care assistance. Wellness applies to the total person: mind, body, and spirit. In facilitating wellness, the caregiving work is not done after a bath, or dressing, or after lunch. The memory impaired person needs activities to stimulate the mind. Music or uplifting words to reach the spirit and stir a memory are all part of facilitating wellness. A memory impaired person retains the right to enjoy the greatest possible degree of wellness. Since that person cannot achieve wellness alone, the caregiver is increasingly important in the role of wellness facilitator.

Learning from the Mistakes of Traditional Caregiving

Family reunions, children's birthday parties, and Valentine's candy in heart boxes are just a few wonderful traditions. These are traditions that link the past with the present as an uplifting, joyful type of connection. On the other hand, there are negative traditions such as child abuse, racial prejudice, and dishonesty with intergenerational links that result in harmful actions from the past to be repeated over and over. In the world of health care for older adults, many attitudes and methods for delivery of care are desperately in need of reform. The primary beliefs behind traditional caregiving suggest that the memory impaired are:

Incapable of self-directed behavior

Disinterested in self-care

Limited in desire to make choices

Unlikely to express a range of emotions

Unable to socialize with others

Only manageable with physical or medical restraints

These negative beliefs support an image of a frail, helpless, powerless person whose only hold on living is sustained by the assistance of others. An assisted care facility or nursing home that allows such negative attitudes to influence the standard of care may be seen as merely "warehousing older adults," rather than giving them good care.

Caregivers working in the traditional systems learn the negative attitudes which result in the tendency to repeat these mistakes:

Treat the impairment not the whole person

Teach or support helplessness and dependence

Limit opportunities for emotional expression

Ignore the value of social interaction

Value custodial care over therapeutic care

Deal with problem behaviors from medical model

Use confrontation instead of communication

Let's examine each of the caregiving mistakes.

Mistake #1: Treat the impairment not the person.

Confusion and memory impairment are conditions a person has, they are not a definition of the total person. In medicine, a person who has cancer is not considered a "cancerous person." Mental health professionals are increasing their own sensitivities in referring to patients. No longer is it acceptable to refer to "the schizophrenic in 505" or "the dementia group." There may be a person who suffers from schizophrenia in room 505 and a current events group for persons with memory impairments. People who face disorders are not disordered people. This is an important difference that needs to be learned by caregivers at all levels, from professionals to para-professionals to health care support services.

Mistake #2: Teach or support helplessness and dependence.

To believe that a memory impaired person is not capable of any self-directed behavior is to act on a false belief. Caregivers who approach persons with this belief are likely to find that their patients become more and more dependent. This is known as "learned helplessness." Teach a person of any age or mental status to depend on others for dressing, feeding, tooth brushing, and other self-care basics and the result is a very dependent person. Helplessness and dependency are strongly connected to depression and loss of personal dignity. Also, skills not practiced are easily forgotten. What seems more practical to do for a memory impaired person is best accomplished by doing with the person. Long after memory fades, a sense of personal dignity remains.

Mistake #3: Limit opportunities for emotional expression.

The ability to feel emotions such as joy, fear, distress, surprise, and security exists from cradle to grave. Trying to limit or deny that memory impaired persons have the full range of human emotions is to deny their humanity. The traditional caretaking approach tries to quiet the memory impaired person with fake caring; "You really aren't upset, everything is fine," "there, there, dear, just be patient," or "Let's stop talking about sad things and cheer up." Restricting emotions only delays or increases the reaction. The memory impaired person needs a safe outlet to express emotions.

Mistake #4: Ignore the value of social interaction.

Persons with memory loss may forget some of their "company manners," however, they can still enjoy social interaction. Merely having all the residents dressed and seated quietly in the day room at the same time is not social interaction. Memory impaired persons have lost certain skills but they never lose the need for positive attention and human contact.

Mistake #5: Value custodial care over therapeutic care.

Many daily tasks must be performed to meet the basic physical needs such as feeding, dressing, showering, and toileting. For all the staff efforts in meeting those needs, too many facilities neglect the emotional, social, and psychological needs of residents. Consider the grim news photos of older persons with sad, lonely expressions slumped over in wheelchairs that line a clean but barren-looking hallway. The custodial care may be up to par, but lacks a humane effort. Traditional caregiving places greater attention to custodial care over the time, training, and awareness needed to attend to the emotional, social, and psychological needs of the memory impaired.

Mistake # 6: Deal with problem behaviors from medical model.

Much of health care clings to the traditional "medical model." This approach waits for a problem to occur, names it, then treats it. A frequent response to a problem is to depend on medications. When the medical model is applied along with traditional caregiving, the caregivers develop attitudes of "learned helplessness" in responding to patients.

If caregivers believe that only medication calms an agitated resident, then they depend on medications instead of one-on-one response to the patient. Problem behaviors may be a way of calling attention to a need; a resident may be too cold, too hot, being bothered by another resident, or needing reorientation in the environment. The staff that depends on medication is stuck in the custodial care philosophy.

Mistake # 7: Use confrontation instead of communication.

What is gained by winning an argument with a memory impaired resident? Nothing. When a person with power (caregiver) confronts, challenges or overpowers a person with less power (i.e., memory impaired resident) the purpose is to gain obedience and control rather than develop communication and trust. In this situation, the caregiver ignores the resident's personal dignity and right to make choices. When the resident is constantly forced to meet the caregiver's schedule for getting dressed, taking a shower and attending certain activities, then the autonomy and basic functioning of the resident is taken away by the staff long before it is lost to the memory impairing condition.

Giving orders or talking down to residents takes less effort than making conversation and really listening to the responses. As memory declines, conversation skills may also decline. However, memory impaired persons try to get the message across with whatever skills they can muster. Caregivers who never take time to tune-in to the communication efforts to each resident in their care find it easier to label residents as "problems" rather than getting to know their needs as persons.

The mistakes and negative beliefs of custodial care blossom where these attitudes are taught and reinforced among the staff at every level of care.

Factors That Perpetuate Traditional Attitudes about Care

The five factors that support traditional caregiving rather than facilitating wellness are:

Factor #1: Institutional Policies and Rules

From an organizational view, the typical assisted care or skilled nursing home is divided into several departments. These territories are usually subdivided according to the scope of job responsibilities; nursing, housekeeping, dietary, and activities. Each department functions according to duties, timetables, and compliance with governmental rules under which the facility is licensed. With so many rules to follow (internal, government, licensing board, etc.), staff can easily be pressed for time. From a time-management viewpoint, the traditional approach says "get it done and get it done fast." Therefore, residents who are less coordinated and move slower are treated like department store mannequins to be dressed, arranged, and set out of the traffic path. Any efforts to encourage a resident to participate in dressing or feeding is abandoned because of time pressures. The more a memory impaired resident gives into "learned helplessness," the greater the amount of time that will eventually be used in providing care for that resident. What seems efficient actually requires more staff time as the resident becomes both discouraged and increasingly dependent.

A division of labor and some areas of specialized training are necessary to make a care facility run smoothly. Unless these "units" or "territories" within the facility work as a team, the organizational structure becomes a way to build walls rather than cooperation. Nursing staff which has no interest in the group therapy programs, a dietary staff merely serving food and trying to avoid conversations with residents, a housekeeping staff trying to get residents to move elsewhere while rooms are being cleaned, or an activities staff only involved with residents during scheduled periods but having no time to chat with those same residents a few hours later in the hallway.

In the above examples, everybody does something, but nobody wants to do anything extra. In this type of caretaking, the custodial duties are done and maybe even rewarded with a high mark at inspection time, but the same facility deserves an "F" for failing to treat memory impaired residents with respect and value as human beings.

Factor #2 Environmental Barriers

Many existing care facilities are placing memory impaired residents into areas that are not designed with consideration for their special needs. Merely placing a locked door on a unit is not enough to make an area suitable for memory impaired residents. Environmental barriers must be corrected in the residents' rooms and common areas that are shared by all residents, families and staff.

The long, hospital green painted corridors without visual cues are like endless tunnels that challenge the navigational abilities of the memory impaired. Sensory deficits are aggravated by decor, object placement, and complexity. As explained in the chapter on modifying the environment, something as simple as a carpet with a small pattern can trigger an obsessive response in a resident who is preoccupied with "trying to pick up the little pieces of paper on the floor." The institutional image is boring to most people and a fearful maze to the memory impaired residents.

Factor # 3 Expectations of Caretaking Staff

No matter how glowing the adjectives used in the promotional brochures, the true expectations of staff are both "taught and caught." In the facility that relies on custodial care techniques, the caretaking method is "taught" by example and possibly by job description. Negative attitudes of the staff toward residents are "caught" by new staff as rapidly as catching a cold germ. Custodial care oriented facilities tend to attract the type of staff members who are not interested in learning about new approaches or building relationships with memory impaired residents. In this setting, staff members give only what is required during their eight hour shifts and nothing more. They leave work after having as little interaction as possible with residents. Caretaking staff are sometimes described by families of residents as rude, cold, insensitive, and mechanical.

Factor # 4 Expectations of Regulatory Authorities

The laws and rules about standards of care for assisted care and skilled nursing homes exist to protect residents. Many regulations must be followed, from safeguarding resident rights to medication reviews, to knowing which chemicals are acceptable for cleaning the showers. Sometimes in the haste to meet a "white glove inspection," concentration on housekeeping and record keeping takes priority over attention to residents' emotional and social needs.

A floor so shiny that it reflects an image like a mirror gets a good grade at inspection as a sign of sanitary conditions. To a memory impaired resident, the glare from a shiny floor distorts the distances and contours of the walkway in a way that is disorienting.

Other rules that are intended to protect resident rights can be so rigid that individual needs are not met. Consider the resident who enjoys holding and caring for a baby doll. If a regulatory agency inspector says that is too "childlike" or "dehumanizing," who wins, the resident or the agency? Another rule demands the "least restrictive environment" for residents. A secured walker or a lap belt to prevent falling from a wheelchair actually make it possible for some residents to be more mobile. Yet a regulatory agency may view these assistance devices as too restrictive if the resident cannot get in and out of the device at will. Looking at the use of these devices during an inspection visit is totally different than watching the resident struggle daily trying to get around in the safest way. Clearly it becomes difficult to balance strict adherence to all the rules with doing what is best for each resident.

Factor # 5 Illusion of Quality Care

From the outside looking in, a "good" facility may be viewed as one where residents are clean, quiet, and not causing problems. Under that definition, it might be assumed that if residents are dressed and sitting in a trance in front of the dayroom television then the staff is doing a "good" job. The flaw in this assumption is that resident passivity is not a sign of contentment, comfort, or satisfaction. Group passivity is more akin to dependency, neglect, and lack of suitable stimulation.

The custodial care methods demand clean halls, tidy rooms, tightly made beds, and residents neatly arranged by rows to blend in with the overall decor. Like all adults, the memory impaired have happy days and sad days, easy to manage days and aggravating days. There is no quality in care that suppresses emotions and denies feelings in the memory impaired.

Wellness Facilitators^SM — the Future of Caregiving

If custodial care and traditional caregiving represent the past, then the *Wellness Facilitator* is the future. Three core beliefs distinguish the Wellness Facilitator from other direct service providers:

1. The memory impaired adult is fully alive, fully interested in human contact, and fully capable of responding as much as possible to a stimulating environment.
2. The memory impaired person's world is what is in sight and at close range.
3. A trained, sensitive Wellness Facilitator really is a "lifeline to care with dignity" for the memory impaired.

Do you share the attitudes of a Wellness Facilitator?
The following is a basic survey of attitudes and beliefs about working with the memory impaired. Take a few minutes to think about these statements and answer each question.

Circle T (true) or F (false).

T F 1. People with Alzheimer's and memory impairments are not able to help in their own care.

T F 2. There is no reason to make conversation with residents since they just forget it later.

T F 3. Screaming, angry residents need to be controlled.

T F 4. Residents are most content when they are calm, quiet, and fed.

T F 5. Nursing and social services are responsible for responding to the needs of the residents, not dietary or housekeeping.

T F 6. Learning one or two ways to use behavior management is enough.

T F 7. Being polite and helpful is enough, you don't have to like working around older adults.

T F 8. Understanding how memory impairment affects residents requires the education and experience of doctors, psychologists, and nurses.

T F 9. Working with the memory impaired is no different than working with other adults in long term care.

T F 10. The purpose of in-service training is to keep going over the basics.

How many statements do you think are true? _____

How many statements do you think are false ? _____

ANSWER KEY: A Wellness Facilitator knows that all 10 statements are FALSE. Consider the brief explanation of each statement as it relates to attitudes about caring for the memory impaired. Evaluate how these answers compare with your training and experience.

1. People with Alzheimer's and memory impairments are not able to help in their own care.
A memory impaired resident may confuse the order of putting on clothing yet still have the ability to get dressed with gentle reminders. Many of the basic self care skills can be performed throughout several stages of memory impairment.

Some tasks need to be divided into single steps. For example, total confusion and acting out may result from placing a resident in front of the sink and saying "brush your teeth." That directive requires a series of small steps performed in a certain order. The frustration of trying to recall the steps, stay in focus, send the motor messages from brain to arms, and self monitor is much too complex. The caregiver may help the resident complete the process by saying and showing one step at a time. Or the caregiver may get toothpaste on the brush, place the brush in the resident's hand, and guide the brush to the teeth before saying and showing, "brush your teeth."

Encouraging each resident to do as much as possible toward self-care is more about building self-esteem than getting everyone's teeth brushed. Guiding and encouraging is facilitating wellness. Taking over and doing for the resident is custodial caretaking.

2. There is no reason to make conversation with residents since they just forget it later.
As previously stated, people with memory impairments are not impaired people. They are people with a disease which includes symptoms of memory loss. Inside they are human beings with all the needs, wants, feelings, fears, and frustrations of any other human being. Caregivers who can't see beyond the impairment are not suited to working with the memory impaired. How sad to miss those "windows of opportunity" that happen without notice when a memory impaired person is really tuned into the here and now. Those moments are crucial to building a rapport with residents and sense of

trust that transcends the impairment. At other times as well, a short verbal exchange in a pleasant, genuine manner when passing a resident in the hallway can make a real difference in the resident's mood.

3. Screaming, angry residents need to be controlled.
Control is a restraint; whether verbal, emotional, or physical. Gaining control over the resident is temporary since the real message sent by the acting out behavior is not received by the caregiver. The resident's needs are not met, so the problem behaviors continue. The Wellness Facilitator will recognize the problem behaviors as the resident's attempt to communicate rather than irritate.

4. Residents are most content when they are calm, quiet, and fed.
Just like the previous statement, this is a negative belief. It's the custodial care oriented staff who is happy when residents are calm, quiet, and fed. However, that does not mean that the residents are happy. Living in such an atmosphere of intimidation and manipulation, the residents have nowhere to go but to withdraw further inside themselves looking for comfort.

5. Nursing and social services are responsible for responding to the needs of the residents, not dietary or housekeeping.
Staying in one's own territory is simple if working on a factory assembly line. It's not easy, or desirable when working with memory impaired residents. A resident does not recall that the blue uniforms are dietary and the white uniforms are nursing. All that the resident sees is being ignored instead of recognized.

Certainly there are tasks specific to the training of each territory within the facility. Yet a few minutes to redirect a resident back toward his or her room can be done by any staff member. Reassurances, comforting, listening, and bringing back appropriate medical help as needed is the job of everyone from the part-time housekeeper to the administrator.

6. Learning one or two ways to use behavior management is enough.
The techniques of behavior management are varied. Some need to be adapted for the memory impaired. New twists on existing behavior management approaches are emerging. To rely on one or two techniques is to barely scratch the surface of possibilities that are so useful in working with the memory impaired.

Ask the facility director of staff development to arrange in-service training on behavior management. Attend any behavioral management programs available from continuing education, universities or agencies on aging. Many techniques are simple to learn and easy to use.

7. Being polite and helpful is enough, you don't have to like working around older adults.

The residents are memory impaired, not stupid. They sense the disdain from a staff member who is not sincere. Being polite and helpful is great in working with any group of people. With the memory impaired, caregivers must have and demonstrate genuine interest and unconditional acceptance of residents. Anything less is not in keeping with facilitating wellness.

8. Understanding how memory impairment affects residents requires the education and experience of doctors, psychologists, and nurses.

All caregivers (family and staff) need a basic knowledge of memory impairment causes, symptoms, and progression. If that knowledge was not part of prior training, it can be acquired through in-service training and reading. In addition to professional training programs, the Alzheimer's Association offers a wealth of free fact sheets and brochures. Call any local Alzheimer's Association office or the national headquarters in Chicago at 312-335-8700.

Consider that a resident sitting in the activity room is feeling chilled but is not able to make the mental connections necessary to ask for a sweater. There is a breakdown in the neuro-transmitters such that the pathway does not move full circle; feeling cold = need sweater = feel warmer. A psychologist may explain how this problem occurs with great detail in full scientific terminology. An observant nursing aide who sees the same resident shivering and sobbing realizes that the resident is sitting in a draft near the door. The aide brings a sweater, shows it, then asks if the resident wants to wear it. The problem is solved without high-tech knowledge.

Graduate school is great, but it's no substitute for caring, observing and listening to the verbal and non-verbal cues that memory impaired residents give in trying to get their needs met.

9. Working with the memory impaired is not really different than working with other adults in long term care.
As part of the aging process, many people experience forgetfulness and mental fatigue more noticeably than in younger years. Illness, nutritional deficiencies, medication, anesthesia, or depression can cause memory problems that are sometimes mistakenly labeled as Alzheimer's. However, these cases have the potential for memory improvement when the causative factor is cured or managed.

The memory impaired elder is very different. The various conditions that result in memory impairment (i.e., Alzheimer's, multi-infarct dementia, etc.) are chronic and progressively worsen with time. Because the effects of memory impairment are unique to each person, no one-size-fits-all treatment approach exists. The caregiver's experience from generalized long term care is useful with adaptations for the memory impaired. To that base of experience, caregivers at all levels (family, professional, and paraprofessional) need continual training in the latest care and management techniques.

As the numbers of the memory impaired population increases, so does research and development of new training resources. This text is just one example of responding to the need for caregiver education.

10. The purpose of in-service training is to keep going over the basics.
Coaches of the most successful sports teams say that they regularly repeat the basics as a foundation for learning new plays. Since the other teams also know the basics, the championship teams are those that add flair and new twists to the classic plays. The same is true in long term care. The basics of long term care for the memory impaired must be taught to new staff and periodically reinforced with experienced staff. That's good, but not enough. Facilitating wellness builds on and expands the basics by reaching for new ideas and techniques to better serve the memory impaired. In-service training is a convenient learning opportunity, not a dull requirement. The staff training director who takes this mission seriously seeks qualified educators from health care professions, educational organizations, and universities. In long term care, the best facilities usually have an

excellent in-service training program. The cost of training is a good investment that compounds daily with renewed interest of staff in delivering quality care.

Remember: behavior follows beliefs. In working with the memory impaired, the caregivers' beliefs about these residents guides the attitudes with which the work is done. The facility with strong beliefs about facilitating wellness brings in like-minded staff to be part of a quality care team.

Reframing Beliefs toward Facilitating Wellness

Caregivers who desire to become Wellness Facilitators can apply a psychological technique called "reframing." Here's an example: think of finding a beautiful landscape painting at a garage sale. The picture is pleasing but something about it is drab. The frame of that picture is too heavy and overpowering. Later when the same picture is cleaned up and placed inside a new, bright, and more stylish frame, the picture takes on a different look. Same picture. New view. That's how reframing works with thought processes. Instead of focusing on the disabilities of the memory impaired, reframe those negative thoughts into positives by actively seeking to identify and encourage the residents' remaining abilities. Support reframed thinking with new information and creative ideas.

A Wellness Facilitator strives toward achieving these goals:

Wellness Goal #1: A safe and secure environment.
Appropriate surroundings for the memory impaired are somewhat different than for other types of nursing home residents. As mentioned earlier in this chapter, memory impaired persons can be easily distressed and disoriented by patterned carpet, shiny floors or frequent furniture moving. Using bright colors and basic symbols at eye level to be used as visual cues are very important. Furnishings must be comfortable and safe (i.e., sturdy chairs with wide arms and tables without glass or sharp edges.) Chapter 6 has more information about customized environmental designs for the memory impaired.

**Wellness Goal #2: Respect every resident's need for privacy
and personal space.**

Many residents share a personal space with a roommate. There is never enough room to bring everything the family is certain that the resident must have. Selecting those special yet safe items that give a room a sense of home is as important to the memory impaired as to anyone else.

Staff must also respect a resident's desire for a "time-out" from the confusion that exists in the common areas or inside the mind by retreating to personal space of the resident's room. This may interfere with a scheduled activity or dinner. After reasonable encouragement to join the group, smart caregivers allow some time for the resident to regain self-control in the privacy of a secure personal space.

**Wellness Goal #3: Encourage decision-making to
enhance self-esteem.**

Like all adults, the memory impaired have likes, dislikes, and needs. Providing opportunities for basic decision-making is an important part of self-esteem. A resident who is involved in self-care becomes more interested in the cooperative response rather than the obstructive response. Try this with something as simple as asking a resident, "would you like to wear the blue sweater or the red sweater?" That is a manageable decision. Opening the closet and asking "what do you want to wear today?" is a confusing, nonproductive decision that leads more to frustration than participation. Keep the decisions basic and offer no more than two choices.

**Wellness Goal #4: Maximize capabilities while supporting
functional deficits.**

As previously stated, doing tasks with the residents takes more time initially but yields a better overall result than doing it for them. According to the recommendations from each resident's physician, the Wellness Facilitator motivates a resident to try harder to reach toward capabilities without demanding responses beyond physical or mental abilities.

Wellness Goal #5: Avoid teaching dependency and learned helplessness.

Genuine concern for the residents is best shown by modeling, motivating, and believing in each individual's potential for independence. This is totally different than the sticky-sweet "there, there, dear, let me help you" attitudes that mold them into helplessness. Wellness Facilitators cheer the effort as much as the result. Memory impaired persons respond to sincere caring much more so than false flattery.

Wellness Goal #6: Learn positive behavioral management techniques as the first response and medication as the last resort in dealing with problem behaviors.

One positive outcome of regulatory agency monitoring is stricter rules that prevent overuse of medication for control of the memory impaired. As a result, all facilities use more behavioral management techniques. Unfortunately, some approaches are little more than intimidation, manipulation, and depersonalization.

Wellness Facilitators prefer the positive techniques of behavioral management that guide the resident toward self-directed behaviors. Another hallmark of Wellness Facilitators is their excitement about learning new positive approaches and sharing what they have learned with others.

Wellness Goal #7: Establish dynamic activities that respond to the physical, emotional and social needs of residents.

Activities for the memory impaired are much more than crafts, coffee clubs, and watching television. A wide range of new possibilities for therapeutic activities are emerging from specialists in music therapy, movement therapy, art therapy, and group psychotherapy. Some of these ideas are adaptable within the skill levels of the present staff while others need input from qualified professionals. The best treatment team plans include a variety of activities or groups that meet at least the most pressing need for each resident's physical, emotional, and social well-being.

Excellent Facilities Seek Wellness Facilitators

The facility looking for Wellness Facilitators and the caregiver looking for a position share the same essential concern. Is there a "goodness of fit" between the facility and the caregiver? A good match means less personnel turnover. High turnover (or change) of employees is expensive and disruptive in any company. In long term care for memory impaired, residents are greatly affected by staff change. Getting to know each resident's abilities and needs is a major part of the job that is as much experienced as taught. Changes in caregivers takes a longer adjustment period for memory impaired residents than for residents in other long term care units.

Correctly responding to the previous survey on attitudes and beliefs gives some indication of a caregiver's heart for working with the memory impaired. Other characteristics of a Wellness Facilitator include:

Genuine interest in caring for older adults

Emotionally stable and self-confident

Strives to leave personal problems at home

Capable of managing stress in healthy ways

Enjoys being part of a quality team

Takes personal pride in work

Willing to learn new techniques

Receives direction positively

Wellness Facilitators have these characteristics plus the training or license appropriate to do their work.

Whether selecting a facility as a place to work or choosing a long term care facility for a memory impaired loved one, the signs of excellence are the same. Facilitating wellness requires a combination of an excellent staff, a quality oriented administration and family involvement.

1. Facilitating wellness seeks to create a homelike environment for the residents.

What motivates residents to feel at home in a facility is one part decor and two parts family atmosphere. While keeping within the regulatory guidelines for cleanliness, the excellent facility makes room for personal touches that give a warm feeling. A fireplace with safe lights (instead of fire) or an outdoor picnic table are familiar family settings. Encourage residents to display favorite photos or non-breakable collectibles (i.e., dolls, postcards, or woodwork).

Even more important are the touches of friendliness that say without words how much the resident is welcome. Helping a new resident feel wrapped into a circle of extended family (staff and other residents) gives security and a sense of belonging to ease the transition. Caregivers are only inside the facility for a certain number of hours weekly. To residents, this facility is their home. Speak of the surroundings like home. "I can walk with you back to your room now." "Please come with me to a sing-a-long in the next neighborhood (unit)." Loyalty to a facility is vague. Loyalty to a neighborhood and the extended family is easier for residents and caregivers to accept.

2. Wellness Facilitators develop a creative activities program for residents.

Activities are not just something to get residents busy while a few more staff take a break. Meaningful activities are important in reducing social isolation, providing sensory stimulation, encouraging movement, and using the natural desire to recall past events in a therapeutic way. Responsive caregivers find activities to fit each resident rather than forcing residents to fit into a specific activity.

More active, physically strong residents can be gathered into a music and movement group with dancing, stretching or walking. Residents with less strength and mobility may be more satisfied with hands-on activities with paints, clay, sand, paper, or smooth wood. Memory impaired residents can do many activities with some extra assistance and slow, one-step-at-a-time directions.

3. Wellness Facilitators work effectively as a team.

Good families work well together and so do effective caregiving teams. Creating the family atmosphere for both residents and workers happens in a facility with real team spirit. Just like baseball players waiting to see where the ball lands, each team member is ready to cover his or her territory. Team members watch the total play and remain ready to help another member. When the team wins, every team member wins. In residential care, a team spirit among staff also means that residents are big winners. A strong team lightens the load for each individual while doubling the efficiency.

4. All staff and families are encouraged to contribute to Treatment Team planning.
Excellent facilities value Treatment Team meetings and encourage caregivers at all levels to share ideas and observations. More than an obligation, these periodic meetings focus attention on the needs, responses, and new approaches tailored to each resident. Treatment Team is not just for the social worker, head nurse and physician. Information and suggestions from every caregiver is vital.

5. A wellness oriented facility recognizes and responds to stress overloads among the staff.
Health care workers are at risk for work-related stress. An extra measure of patience and gentleness is required in caring for the memory impaired. Add to that expectation the other demands of life (i.e., family, relationships, finances) and a caregiver's stress load quickly becomes very heavy. Facilitating wellness among the staff means to recognize this risk and offer help. That help may be with a stress management group for caregivers, exercise program, relaxation training, or counseling. Guiding the caregiver toward healthy ways of releasing stress reduces absences and accident potential while increasing team efficiency.

Wellness Facilitators are Pioneers

Do these wellness goals sound hard to reach? Consider that the entire field of gerontology is the new kid on the block in both medicine and psychology. There is much to learn and discover about elder care. Wellness Facilitators for the memory impaired are true pioneers. Catch that spirit of adventure and pride. Whether preparing food service, transporting a resident to physical therapy, conducting a group or helping reluctant residents through the dreaded shower time, what is learned in facilities today contributes toward setting the standard of quality care for future years.

Glossary

Ageism   A demeaning attitude which results in discrimination against people because of their age.

Agitation   Extreme distress or discomfort that results in aggressive behaviors such as hitting, biting, pushing, cursing, or otherwise attempting to channel negative feelings outwardly toward other persons or things.

Abnormal memory function   Occurs when any portion (long term or short term) of the memory functioning ceases to operate or be accessible on demand.

Agnosia   A neurologic deficit that involves the loss of sensory perceptions necessary to accurately identify a person, place, or object.

Alzheimer's disease   The most commonly known form of dementia with a steady decline in cognitive processing necessary for abstract and rational thinking, progressive memory loss, difficulty with spoken or written language, decreased impulse control, and loss of social skills.

Alzheimer's Association   An international organization dedicated to providing resources, family support, education, nursing home care, respite care and autopsy assistance. The association publishes a newsletter and books for health care professionals, sponsors research, and monitors public policy. The mission is well summarized by its motto, "Someone to stand by you."

Aphasia   A neurologic deficit that results in loss of language skills including the ability to read and write.

Apraxia   A neurologic deficit that is evidenced in a gradual or sudden decline in motor skills.

Cognitive decline   A notable or progressive reduction in prior levels of thought, reasoning, and memory.

Cognitive impairment   Due to cognitive decline, a person with this condition is impaired, or not capable of functioning at a level that existed prior to the debilitating condition.

Combativeness   Efforts to physically repel contact by engaging in kicking, hitting, biting, punching, cursing, or other actions that can be dangerous to the caregiver.

Confusion   An interruption of the memory process resulting in temporary or episodic disorientation sufficient to cause difficulty functioning within the environment.

Custodial care   Care for the physical body with minimal consideration for nurturing the emotional or spiritual needs.

Dementia   A brain disease that is characterized by loss of cognitive processing severe enough to interfere with activities of daily living, reasoning, thinking, and behaviors.

Depression   A single episode or a recurrent problem that is evidenced by a pervasive disturbance of mood with feelings of helplessness and hopelessness.

Environmental design   This is an important element in creating a healthy, stimulating living space for the memory impaired which will support functioning and reduce mobility risks.

Hallucination   Often accompanies agnosia (loss of sensory perceptions) and is characterized by claims of sensory contact with people or things that are not verifiable .

Harmful stress   Any stress that is negative, painful, sad, oppressive, or overwhelming.

Incontinence   Inability to control urination or defecation.

Irreversible dementia   Progressively declining memory impairment results from irreversible conditions such as vascular dementia, Alzheimer's disease, HIV related dementia, other types of dementia, head injury, and chemical poisoning.

Learned helplessness   Whether ignoring cries for help or being so helpful as to suppress efforts at self-care, the resident is taught that being incapable is expected. Thus over time, the resident "learns helplessness" and becomes dependent on caregivers.

Locomotion   The ability to move from place to place under own power or direction.

Long-term memory   The portion of the memory that is a permanent storage center with unlimited capacity.

Medical model   Waits for a problem to occur, names the problem, then treats the problem. Preventative care is not significant in this model.

Memory   A process of receiving information, storing information, and retrieving information.

Memory impairment   A chronic interruption of the memory process resulting in permanent disorientation to person, place and time that is evidenced by a progressive decline in short-term and long-term memory. This condition may be temporary if resulting from a reversible dementia such as depression, anesthesia, medication, extreme fatigue, nutritional deficiencies, sensory deficits, medical conditions, or grief.

Multi-infarct dementia   Distinguished by a series of mini-strokes (infarcts) that cause damage to areas of the brain. Cognitive and skill declines are rapid and erratic rather than the slow progressive decline seen in persons with Alzheimer's disease.

Multi-modal   Based on a concept defined by Arnold Lazarus in which the evaluation of an individual is made with consideration to all of these aspects; behavior, affect, sensation, imagery, cognition, interpersonal relationships, and diet or drugs.

Non-verbal communication   Transmitting messages with facial gestures, movements, and other bodily responses.

Paranoia   Inability to distinguish reality from perceptions or beliefs of pending harm.

Problem behavior   Any behavior that interrupts functioning in a way that endangers the safety of the individual or other persons in the environment.

Productive stress   Any stress that gives a person the extra drive, motivation, anticipation, or energy to be more creative in positive, healthy ways.

Reminiscence   Recalling memories as part of an aging person's natural desire to review the past. When used as a therapeutic modality, reminiscence is an established technique for individual therapy and geriatric groups.

Repetitive actions   Ongoing movements without a direct purpose which can be soothing to the memory impaired or can be actions of self-harm.

Reversible dementia   Some memory impairment that appears similar to dementia may result from conditions that are subject to improvement, such as depression, anesthesia, medication, extreme fatigue, nutritional deficiencies, sensory deficits, medical conditions, or grief.

Sensory stimulation   An effort to help the memory impaired reconnect with their five senses through the use of objects, activities, and environmental design.

Sensory deficits   Loss or diminished abilities in any of the five senses (touch, taste, smell, hearing, vision).

Sexually inappropriate   For a memory impaired person, this type of behavior typically includes taking off clothing at the wrong time or place, masturbating, or aggressive touching of others. The memory impaired forget social rules of behavior and sexual expression.

Short-term memory   The portion of the memory that is the active process operating in the here and now.

Stages of memory impairment   In this text, the stages are explained according to the seven levels of cognitive decline as defined by the Global Deterioration Scale.

Stress   A demand oriented response with notable physical and emotional arousal.

Traditional care   An effort to relate with residents which is often overpowered by custodial needs. This approach is characterized by focusing on disabilities rather than abilities.

Vascular dementia   same as multi-infarct dementia

Wellness Facilitators   Skilled, sensitive, positive-oriented people who work in their unique areas of health care providing services to memory impaired adults.

Stages of Care

Families make a series of decisions about caregiving for the memory impaired from among these options.

Home Health Care supports the family caregiver by providing services as needed for skilled nursing, home health aides, home-making and other specialized services.

Assisted Care Living is just what is required to meet personal needs and perform activities of daily living (i.e., bathing, dressing, eating, ambulation, or taking medication). Generally this level of care is provided in an ALF adult congregate living center. ALF's can be small (4-6 residents) or large multi-story complexes with hundreds of residents.

Intermediate Care includes residential care with occasional skilled nursing assistance and rehabilitative services that can only be provided by, or under supervision of, licensed health care personnel.

Skilled Care is more commonly known as a "nursing home" or SNF -skilled nursing facility. This residential care includes daily skilled nursing and rehabilitative services that can only be provided by, or under supervision of, licensed health care personnel. The care may be custodial (long term illness or disability) or restorative (returning patient to condition of health as existed before the illness or injury).

DSCU is a dementia specific care unit, found in residential care facilities. These units have specially trained personnel, secure boundaries and activities to stimulate dementia patients to function as independently as possible.

Organizations

The following organizations provide valuable resources for family
and staff caregivers including brochures, books, fact sheets,
hotlines, and referrals.

Alzheimer's Association
919 North Michigan, Suite 1000
Chicago, IL 60611-1676
(800)272-3900   (312) 335-5776   (312) 335-8882 (TDD)

Alzheimer's Disease Education & Referral Center
PO Box 8250
Silver Springs, MD 20907-8250
(800) 438-4380

American Speech-Language-Hearing Association
10801 Rockville Pike
Rockville, MA 20852
(800) 638-8255

Help for Incontinent People, Inc.
PO Box 544
Union, SC 29379
(800) 252-3337   (803)579-7900

National Family Caregivers Association
9223 Longbranch Parkway
Silver Spring, MD 20901-3642
(301) 949-3638

National Institute on Aging Information Center
PO Box 8057
Gaithersburg, MD 20898-8057
(800) 222-2225

Resources

AARP Publications Catalog
PO Box 51040, Station R, Washington, DC 20091
(202) 434-2277

American Association of Music Therapy
PO Box 80012, Valley Forge, PA 19484
(610) 265-4006

Eldergames, Inc. (1993)
11710 Hunters Lane, Rockville, MD 20852
(301) 984-8336 or (800) 637-2604

Eldersong Newsletter
Eldersong Publications, Inc.
PO Box 74, Mr. Airy, MD 21771
(301) 829-0533   Subscription: $15 per year or $26 for 2 years.

Geriatric Resources
Catalog of books, equipment, and. caregiver teaching materials.
PO Box 239, Radium Springs, NM 88054-0239
(800) 359-0390   Fax (505) 524-0254

National Association for Music Therapy
8455 Colesville Road, Suite 930, Silver Spring, MD 20910
(301) 589-3300

National Institute on Aging
Free list of publications on aging and health.
(800) 222-2225 or www.nih.gov.nia

Sharing the Caring (video)
National Adult Daycare Services Association,
(800) 867-2755. Order #PSA-1. $35.00

Wise Now Newsletter
Better Directions, Inc.
PO Box 752, Melbourne, FL 32902
(407) 724-5767. Subscription $29.95

References

Butler, R.N., Lewis, M.I., Sunderland, T. (1991). *Aging and mental health: positive psychosocial and biomedical approaches.* (4th ed.) Columbus, OH: Charles E. Merrill.

Hinrichsen, G.A. (1992). Recovery and relapse from major depressive disorder in the elderly. *American Journal of Psychiatry,* 149, 1575-1579.

Lazarus, A. A. (1976). *Multi-modal behavior therapy.* New York: Springer

Lovelace, E.A. (1990). Basic concepts in cognition and aging. In E.A. Lovelace (Ed.), *Aging and cognition: mental processes, self-awareness and interventions* (pp.1-28).Vancouver: Elsevier Science Publishers.

Meichenbaum, D. & Cameron, R. (1974). The clinical potential of modifying what clients say to themselves. In M.J. Mahoney & C.E. Thoreson, *Self-Control: power to the person.* New York: Wadsworth, Inc.

National Institutes of Health. (1991). *NIH Consensus Development Conference: Diagnosis and treatment of depression in late life,* 9, no.3, 1-22

National Institutes of Health. (1988). Consensus development conference statement. *Journal of American Geriatric Society,* 36, 342-7.

Recommended Reading

Bowlby, C. (1993). *Therapeutic activities for persons disabled by Alzheimer's disease and related disorders.* Rockville, MD: National Health Publishers.

Brantley, E. (1995). *Designing for Alzheimer's.* New York: John Wiley Publications.

Burnside, I.M. & Schmidt, M. (1994). *Working with older adults: group process and techniques.* (3rd ed.) Boston: Jones & Bartlett.

Cohen, D. (1995). *Caring for your aging parents: a planning and action guide.* New York: G.P. Putnam.

Coons, D.H. (ed.) (1991). *Specialized dementia care units.* Baltimore, MD: Johns Hopkins University Press.

Doukas, D. & Reichel, W. (1993). *Planning for uncertainty: a guide to living wills and other advance directives for health care.* Baltimore, MD: Johns Hopkins University Press.

Edwards, A. (1994). *When memory fails: helping the Alzheimer's and dementia patient.* New York: Plenum.

Erwin, K.T. (1996). *Group techniques for aging adults.* Washington, DC: Taylor & Francis.

Gallo, J.J., Reichel, W., & Andersen, L.M. (1995). *Handbook of geriatric assessment.* Aspen Publishers: Gaithersburg, MD.

Haight, B.K. & Webster, J.D. (1995). *The art and science of reminiscing.* Washington, DC: Taylor & Francis.

Hoffman, S.B. & Platt, C.A. (1991). *Comforting the confused.* New York: Springer Publishing Company.

Lakin, M. (1995). *When someone you love has Alzheimer's Disease.* New York: Dell Publishing.

Mace, N.L. & Rabins, P.V. (1991). *The 36 hour day (rev. edition).* Baltimore, MD: Johns Hopkins University Press.

McGowin, D. (1993). *Living in the labrinth: a personal journal through the maze of Alzheimer's.* New York: Delacorte Press.

Schelle, J.F. (1991). *Managing urinary incontinence in the elderly.* New York: Springer Publishing Company.

Waters, E.B. & Goodman, J. (1990). *Empowering older adults.* San Francisco, CA: Jossey-Bass.

Zarit, S.H., Orr, N.K., & Zarit, J.M. (1985). *The hidden victims of Alzheimer's Disease.* New York: New York University Press.

Zarit, S.H., Pearlin, L.I., Schaie, K.W. (eds.) (1993). *Caregiving systems: informal and formal helpers.* Hillsdale, NJ: Lawrence Erlbaum Associates.

Books that help children understand Alzheimer's

Bahr, M. (1992). *The memory box.* Morton Grove, IL: Whitman. (Grandfather who has Alzheimer's Disease prepares a memory box with his grandson.)

Guthrie, D. (1986). *Grandpa doesn't know it's me.* New York: Human Sciences Press. (A child observes her grandfathers' unusal behaviors and tries to understand.)

McCrea, J. (1992). *Talking with children and teens about Alzheimer's disease: a question and answer guidebook for parents, teachers, and caregivers.* Pittsburgh, PA: Generations Together.

Poatacke, R. (1993). *Always Gramma.* New York: Putnam Press. (Impressions of a young child about grandmother's confusion and forgetfulness.)

Whitelaw, N. (1991). *A beautiful pearl.* Morton Grove, IL: Whitman. (Alghough Grandmother's mental capacities are declining, she prepares a special birthday gift that her granddaughter will always remember.)

Index

Abnormal memory functioning, 5
Activity changes, 121-124
Agnosia, 22-23
Alzheimer's disease, 7, 11-12, 15, 31-33
Anesthesia, 7, 8
Aphasia, 22-23
Apraxia, 22-23
Assessment Summary Report, 51, 60-61
Behavior Checklist, 51, 58-59
Chemical poisoning, 7, 12-13
Communication, #1 principle, 68
Communication, nonverbal, 67-68
Communication, verbal, 65-66
Confusion, defined, 6
Decor choices, 84-87
Depression, 7, 8
Economic changes, 117-120
Exterior design, 88-89
Extreme fatigue, 7, 9
Geriatric Depression Scale, 51, 56-57
Grief, 7, 11
Global Deterioration Scale, 18, 19
HIV-related dementia, 7, 12
Head injury, 7, 12
Identification, 87-88
Interior spaces, 80-83
Location changes, 124-126
Long term memory, 4

Medication, 7, 9
Medical conditions, 7, 10-11
Memory, basic definition, 3, 13
Memory impairment, basic definition, 7, 13
Mini-Mental State Exam, 51, 54-55
Multi-infarct dementia, 12, 15, 16
Nutritional deficiencies, 7, 10
Personal safety, 90-91
Problem Behavior(s), 24-27, 94-112
Relationship changes, 115-117
Sensory deficits, 7, 10
Short Portable Mental Status Quesionnaire, 51-53
Short term memory, 3-4
Stages of memory impairment, 15-17
Stress, 138-150
Stress, harmful, 140
Stress, productive, 140
Vascular dementia, 7, 12
Wellness facilitators, 151-153, 159-161, 165-170
Zarit Burden Interview, 130-131